Research for Health Policy

Research for Health Policy

Erica Bell

Deputy Director,
University Department of Rural Health,
University of Tasmania,
Australia

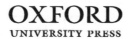

OXFORD
UNIVERSITY PRESS

OXFORD
UNIVERSITY PRESS

Great Clarendon Street, Oxford ox2 6DP

Oxford University Press is a department of the University of Oxford.
It furthers the University's objective of excellence in research, scholarship,
and education by publishing worldwide in

Oxford New York

Auckland Cape Town Dar es Salaam Hong Kong Karachi
Kuala Lumpur Madrid Melbourne Mexico City Nairobi
New Delhi Shanghai Taipei Toronto

With offices in

Argentina Austria Brazil Chile Czech Republic France Greece
Guatemala Hungary Italy Japan Poland Portugal Singapore
South Korea Switzerland Thailand Turkey Ukraine Vietnam

Oxford is a registered trade mark of Oxford University Press
in the UK and in certain other countries

Published in the United States
by Oxford University Press Inc., New York

British Library Cataloguing in Publication Data

Data available

Library of Congress Cataloging in Publication Data

Data available

Typeset in Minion by Cepha Imaging Private Ltd., Bangalore, India
Printed in Great Britain
on acid-free paper by
the MPG Books Group, Bodmin and King's Lynn

ISBN 978–0–19–954933–7

10 9 8 7 6 5 4 3 2 1

There are other reasons why things do not happen, reasons
that will not disappear in the light of advancing knowledge alone.
Well-defined, though narrowly based, economic interests will
be threatened by any serious efforts to act on the non-medical
determinants of health. Lavis et al. remind us of this reality, quoting
the eminent American philosopher Homer Simpson: "Just because
I don't care doesn't mean I don't understand."

Evans RG, Stoddart GL. Consuming research, producing policy?
Am J Public Health 2003; 93(3): 378.

University training for researchers probably needs to be rethought so
that they bring a whole range of techniques to policy-making . . .
I don't believe that our education systems are matching the rapid
global changes . . . there are some practices that are prevailing from
people who have been trained in a certain way and are imparting
the same knowledge, so that we're not developing our professional
thinking outside of what we have been used to and we are comfortable
with. And it is hard work to change: it is hard work sometimes to do
anything other than what you've been traditionally taught.

(health agency CEO)

Acknowledgements

Twenty-two policy-makers involved in the management of health services at national surgeon-general, state director-general, and regional authority CEO levels, consented to be interviewed for this book. They came from 11 countries: United Kingdom, United States, Canada, Australia, New Zealand, Singapore, Hong Kong, Denmark, Switzerland, Sweden, and Norway. Without them this book would not have been possible.

The project was partly funded by the University Department of Rural Health under a grant from the Australian government Department of Health and Ageing. Thanks are also owed to the staff of the Hobart Clinical Library at the University of Tasmania for their unfailing generosity with the difficult task of gathering together evidence from diverse sources.

Particular thanks are owed to the international leaders in these areas—Charles Ragin, Huw Davies, and Deborah Stone—for offering writings that challenged and extended my thinking. I also thank those many other scholars whose publications I have cited in this book, and hope that I have done your work justice.

Acknowledgement should also be made of the hundreds of attendees at my workshops and presentations on research methods for policy and practice. Their passion for the subject of how to produce more socially useful research was infectious and gave me the idea of writing this book. Siobhan Harpur, Director, State-Wide System Development, at Tasmania's Department of Health and Human Services, gave me very helpful feedback on the usefulness of this book for policy-making.

My thanks must also include my partner Bastian Seidel, for his continuing support. This book is dedicated to Nick Bell.

Contents

Introduction

The approach used in this book and its rationale

Many of us in health want to influence and ideally change health policy. Whether we are consumer advocates, health practitioners, staff of professional associations, health services administrators, government department workers, or university researchers, we are asking 'How can we deliver evidence that shapes health policy?'

The challenges of delivering powerful evidence are shared across health sectors and national borders, and the demands they place on research methods are generic, cross-disciplinary ones. Internationally, it seems we have reached a cross-road in research for health policy. Climate change and the challenges of sustainable development, the election of Barack Obama on a platform of ethical, evidence-based policy-making, and the global economic meltdown have all changed the political and environmental conditions shaping health policy. Across different health specialities, policy-makers are facing big challenges that demand holistic research evidence that speaks to new models of health and ways of policy-making. Researchers know that if we want to deliver better evidence to health policy-makers we need more than what our research training has taught us with its emphasis on traditional classical experimental techniques and the standard qualitative methods. Many in the health field feel ill-prepared for this brave new world of policy-making: we feel uncertain about the styles of evidence that will be effective; perhaps unconvinced research can make a difference. On the other hand, policy-makers can feel that researchers are unreceptive to the idea that their contexts demand particular styles of evidence-making rarely taught in university courses. This book tries to bridge that policy-research divide.

Of course, policy-making is not always influenced by research evidence. When it is, the research genres involved can be quite different: for example, the results of systematic reviews in academic journals, clinical practice guidelines, or studies commissioned by government or other agencies under specific terms of reference. *Research for Health Policy* focuses upon the doing of research for policy. It is sometimes assumed that getting better research-policy transfer is about getting policy-makers to appreciate the value of scholarly research—the 'enlightenment' approach to policy-makers. Yet the challenges of research-policy transfer are also about better understanding the kinds of knowledge, language forms, and evidence-making that has been developed specifically to meet policy decision-making needs. Relatively little is known about the 'nuts and bolts' practices of professional policy-making researchers. Attention to the practices of these researchers—which I have daringly called 'policy-relevant research' in this book—can help build knowledge of how to variously influence policy-makers.

This book aims to equip the reader with the 'hands on' knowledge, skills, and attitudes needed to deliver research for health policy, in the government, not-for-profit, and private sectors. It focuses on describing research for health policy in a heuristic, practice-based way. It tries to help the reader to develop the blend of strategic people skills, methodological inventiveness, research entrepreneurship, creative design, and policy writing know-how that is critical to delivering useful research evidence for health policy.

The book does this by giving the reader both conceptual understandings and practical procedural information about research for policy-making. It focuses on generic or generally applicable, non-technical skills rather than building specialist knowledge and skills in any one area of research for health policy. It also gives the reader step-by-step practical advice on each stages of delivering policy-relevant research: the preparatory stage of deciphering often unwritten policy challenges; the review stage, including local experience and international models; designing and implementing research methods for health policy, including community consultations; delivering the policy 'story' or presenting a persuasive policy argument; writing sound policy options, and managing the dissemination of research in ways that maximize its take-up. In so doing, this book focuses not simply on describing the genre of policy-relevant research as it is often found in reports for policy-makers. Much space is also given to describing and reinventing new methodologies in the scholarly literature from different disciplines that can help develop the rigour and usefulness of this genre. In this way, *Research for Health Policy* is not about defending a particular definition of, or approach to, doing research for health policy. It is more about using a wide range of sources to re-imagine what research for health policy could be.

Accordingly, there are two assertions underpinning the approach in this book:

1 That the traditional quantitative and qualitative research methodologies often used to deliver evidence to policy-makers in health need re-inventing, in ways that are informed by pragmatic methodological innovations in the

scholarly literature, including disciplines beyond the health sciences, where the usefulness of research is being hotly debated in quite different ways.

2 That there is an emerging genre of policy-relevant research that deserves an effort of study because it has not yet been properly identified, theorized, and described.

The first assertion is possibly controversial to some policy-makers because it implies that there are important methodological developments coming out of university research contexts that challenge them to extend the styles of evidence-making with which they are familiar. The second assertion is possibly controversial to some in university research contexts because it implies that there is an emerging research genre not necessarily produced or always well-understood in those contexts, despite so much scholarly research into policy. The book offers many references from different disciplines to support these two assertions.

However different its approach may be to some health policy scholarship, this book reflects the commitment of many scholars to supporting democratic styles of policy-making. That is, the aim of this book is to support those researchers who wish to act as active agents for democratic policy-making processes, by acknowledging the complexity of those processes and the styles of evidence-making needed for them.

If the two assertions underpinning this book have a scholarly evidence base, they are also creatures of the author's location in a historical moment, culture, and generation. First, they emerge from the author's practical experience as a government policy research manager and consultant, health academic, mentor, and workshop presenter in this area. The assumption that university courses incorporating the usual research methods prepare researchers for policy-making contexts becomes very questionable if you have had to teach graduates a particular genre of research you yourself had to learn for public policy-making, and if you have heard policy-makers say how hard it is to find researchers who understand (or are even receptive to learning about) the different styles of evidence-making they need. The idea that this policy-relevant genre needs development in health in particular, using the new methodologies coming out of different disciplines, seems logical if you are a creature of the electronic information explosion age that is creating a whole new generation of discipline-jumping multi-disciplinarians. The electronic information age allows researchers to integrate large amounts of information across disciplines in ways that have potential for not only problem-solving but also questioning the discipline-based assumptions informing the definition of the problem. In such an age it seems natural to ask 'If we really want to deliver quality evidence for health policy-makers why don't we make better use of the new methodologies emerging in other disciplines?'

Throughout this book, three different kinds of sources are used to offer the reader ideas about ways of doing policy-relevant research:

1 The international scholarly literature in health and other disciplines, relevant to specific content areas of health policy, processes of policy-making, and research methods for policy.

2 The international literature outside scholarly journals and monographs, including case studies from different countries, sectors, content areas, and contexts, illustrating how to do research for health policy.

3 A purposive sample of interviews conducted for this book with leading health policy decision-makers at surgeon-general, director-general, and CEO level, in different sectors, in the United Kingdom, United States, Canada, Australia, New Zealand, Singapore, Hong Kong, Denmark, Switzerland, Sweden, and Norway, about what they see as the generic attributes of powerful research evidence for changing policy.

The book also includes discussion of practical tools and exercises, hypotheticals, guides and references aimed at building the reader's mastery. It is designed to work as a resource for graduate students and professionals who want to learn more about how to shape health policy, whether they are based in universities, government, or the not-for-profit, and private enterprise sectors. Accordingly, it assumes knowledge of the fundamentals of research methods taught in undergraduate courses. It is not a textbook because it offers many new techniques and approaches to health research, drawing on a disparate body of established and new primary evidence. As such, it aims to offer an original contribution to the field of health policy by reconceptualizing and reinventing research practice.

This book should also be of value to graduates studying policy or doing research for policy in disciplines and portfolios beyond health. Policy-relevant research in health places some distinctive challenges on the researcher's strategic, writing, and methodological skills. However, learning about those challenges can help researchers beyond health acquire the generic research skills important to meeting policy challenges that cut across discipline and portfolio boundaries. As such, this book is for all those who want to build their knowledge of doing research for policy-makers.

Chapter 1

What changes health policy?

Overview

The task of using evidence to influence health policy-makers is best approached with the benefit of insight into what changes policy. This chapter offers conceptual and practical understandings of how health policy works and what changes it.

Defining policy

What is policy? One working definition of policy is as follows:

> Policies are the set of forces within the control of the policymakers that affect the structure and performance of the system of interest. Loosely speaking, a policy is a set of actions taken by an administration to control the system, to help solve problems within it or caused by it, or to obtain benefits from it.[1] (p. 6)

The 'policy problem' is a definition of what needs to be overcome to achieve such policy ends. Thus, it is frequently a set of tensions, barriers, and challenges associated with a particular policy goal.

More complex definitions of policy using different typologies are available in scholarly literature. However, they can be the subject of much argument. Drawing on the work of other researchers, Lavis et al. define

- functional policies to do with the roles or services for a society or sector
- intentional policies to do with statements of purposes or goals
- population-focused policies to do with statements and actions that target a particular group
- programmatic policies that relate to a package of related policies.[2, 3]

However, Lavis et al. also acknowledge that they could not find a commonly accepted typology of healthcare policy. They further defined functional categories of policy important to the healthcare sector in terms of

- jurisdictional and/or governance policy to do with establishing jurisdictional responsibilities and accountabilities

- financial policy to do with financing, funding, and remuneration decisions about support services

- delivery policy to do with how, by whom, and in what settings services will be delivered and accessed

- programme policy to do with the content of services that will be provided for whom.[2]

Such typologies focus on what policy does or what it is about. However, policy can also be conceptualized in terms of the stages or processes of policy-making: in terms of agenda setting, policy formulation, and policy implementation.[4]

Policy-makers can be contrasted with practitioners who implement (and interpret) policy. In practice the two categories of 'policy' and 'practice' are not separate. For example, a review of health research and policy-making identified three kinds of policy-making: governance/legislative policy-making; service/administrative policy-making; and practice/clinical policy-making.[4] This reflects the different kinds of roles that policy-makers can have: legislators, bureaucrats, clinical health service administrators, and so on.

Policy-makers are parties to a complex process that can also be defined in terms of its level of operation. Policy operates at the micro (local community), meso (regional or state), and macro (national or international) levels. For example, at the macro level, official European Union (EU) decisions may shape what happens in health policy and thus service delivery in Britain and other EU countries.[5] The levels of policy-making may be connected and disconnected in different ways:

> One of the things we talk about is whole of government approaches, inter-sectoral collaboration, the silo mentality, lack of coordination—and we talk about it in the layers of central structures of an organisation and across government, then we will refer to the regional structures and local. None of us have ever really commissioned work around what are the effective points of engagement of the three tiers of state, regional and local, where is it most effective and what makes it effective? We know anecdotally that people who work in a country town in human service agencies tend to gather together in order to have a mutual way of solving some very complex problems. They work without those constraints because they're much more practical in the way they do their work. On the other hand regional directors tend to be much more guarded and have a sense that things need to be done but don't have the authority to make some of the decisions that they would like to make, but tend to seek in many instances clarification from the centre. And in the central agencies, the talk is about whole of government approaches but they often don't practise it.
>
> (health agency CEO)

Policy can also be defined in terms of how it is expressed: explicit statements and guidelines or implicit expectations, and both can shape practice powerfully.

Policy can be made directly or indirectly or even unintentionally. For example, an EU law or treaty article may lead to unplanned changes to health policy that arise from litigation.[5]

Policy can also be defined in terms of the different kinds of agencies that can be involved in policy-making: from government to non-government agencies and also professional and health consumer bodies. Different policy settings will shape the characteristics of policy-makers and the way policy is made. For example, it has been argued that the short-term contracts and high job mobility of National Health Service (NHS) managers can work against the development of partnerships and ongoing dialogue with researchers.[6]

Key ideas

In practice, a useful typology of healthcare policy is one that works for the context in which policy must be made.

This book focuses on the research for public policy-making rather than the research for policies that relate to institutional or professional practice. However, much that this book offers applies to other kinds of policy.

Models of research in policy change

. . . the legislators and the governor want data, they want numbers, they want as accurate information as they can get. But then when that is given to them they also depend and rely a lot on the political environment—that changes when the elected officials change and when people in other positions change. So you have the data as the foundation and then you use the political side of policy-making, depending on who the players are. It's a very dynamic process.

(health agency CEO)

It is not the purpose of this book to detail theoretical models of policy-making: only an outline is given here. There is a large body of literature with diverse agendas on what health reforms ought to be made and how policy analysis should be done.[7] However, in the absence of a systematic, persuasive evidence base for how health policy itself is actually made, this book canvasses a range of ideas that can help researchers develop policy-relevant research approaches.

Weiss identified different ways in which evidence can be used in policy-making: in direct ways in a knowledge-driven model; as part of a rational problem-solving effort that gathers evidence; as one of a range of different interacting considerations that may be strategic and political; as part of a political effort to justify a pre-determined position; and as part of a delaying tactic.[8]

Drawing on the work of Weiss,[8] in *What Works? Evidence Based Policy and Practice in Public Services* Nutley and Webb identify different uses of research related to models of policy change.[9] The models include:

1 a simplistic rational model of policy-making in which evidence feeds directly into the policy-making process, problem-solving as if irrationality and interests did not also play a major role.

2 an incremental or pluralist model of policy-making which sees it as formed in a piecemeal fashion, and in which research can be used in different inter-active ways by different interest groups and players to reach consensus.

Thus, evidence may be seen to play a different role depending on the model of policy-making that is used. Actually, research is probably used in many different ways in most of the complex policy-making systems in which policy networks operate to shape policy change.[9]

It can be easily seen that these different models of policy change are based on particular world views. For example, the rational model of policy-making is consistent with positivist, biomedical approaches to decision-making. It assumes a linear process in which the problem is identified, policy is formu-lated, implemented, and evaluated. That is, it assumes that policy goals can be known and policy options can be selected that, on the basis of extant evidence, best fit these goals.[10]

However, in real world policy-making, the policy problem, solutions, and evidence can be shifting, poorly defined and ill-aligned. Politically conditioned values, culture, and historical factors act to shape the choices that must be made. There are certainly many examples of policy decisions that have been made by introducing and abolishing change, apparently without evidence of any kind, purely for political reasons.[11] The incremental model of policy-making accounts for this by focussing on the process of bargaining and adjustment among different interests.[10]

Lavis et al. offer three groups of factors that shape healthcare policy, devel-oped from their study of Canadian policy-makers:

◆ ideas: not just from research, but from other kinds of information, as well as the values of legislators, stakeholders, and the wider public

◆ interests: of stakeholders, legislators, and policy advisors

◆ institutions: past policies, the nature (openness) of the policy-making process, timeframes relevant to the policy-making process, and the nature of approvals needed for policy.[2]

Clearly, before policy can be implemented, many different factors need to be working favourably. Often, the policy must be feasible, legitimated and supported, in different ways. For example, 'feasibility' can include technical, financial, and administrative considerations.[10, 12] 'Support' for a particular policy option refers not simply to explicit support but also the many ways in which different stakeholders unknown to researchers can indirectly support a particular policy direction in different ways though a complex web of policy networks. These dynamics can be observed within organizations:

> . . . at the macro level we have pretty good systems in several different areas for advising the government in the publicly funded system, where they should invest their dollars especially when it comes to either new or expensive therapies. But what about the micro level? What about inside our organisation? The problem here is that we provide care based on the parameters that drive the publicly funded system, and encourage the provincial government to set those parameters based on the best evidence of what works and what doesn't. We generally don't do that ourselves within the hospital networks that I run . . . if there is a new expensive procedure we will evaluate the evidence that technical experts—be they doctors, surgeons—bring to the table. But we will usually say, 'Look you can't really do that without specific funding since these things are usually more expensive.' We will help make the advocacy case through the funding authorities . . . So at the micro level we're probably more working to facilitate information transfer to the funding stakeholder than we are to make funding decisions constantly ourselves. We do have some roles where we do a field valuation or a very small pilot of a totally new procedure, and there we will sometimes swallow the expense—but we try to avoid that as often as we can.
>
> (health agency CEO)

There are many such real world limitations that qualify available models of policy change. Models of policy change do not always properly account for how specific structures work in particular contexts; for example, the ways in which the configuration and application of state authority can actually work against policy objectives, as suggested by debates about health policy.[13] Nor do scholarly models of policy change account for the evidence from at least one survey of policy-makers published by the Cabinet Office of the UK Government that change can be often led 'from the top' by particular ministers and the most senior members of the public service.[14]

The role of community interest groups can also bring extraordinary complexity to policy-making. Mechanic argues in his recent work *The Truth about Health Care: Why Reform is not Working in America* that achieving consensus and implementing change has been very difficult in that country because American values, culture, and ideologies shape the nature of the healthcare market and make it resistant to change.[15] In contrast, Majone argues that many conceptualizations of policy change place too much emphasis on the role of external economic and political forces shaping policy-makers. He argues that much policy change is the result of the often unanticipated effects of previous public policy processes and their consequences rather than deliberate choice by policy-makers.[16]

Available models of policy change also do not always account for how a single focusing event or sudden exceptional experience (such as a hospital error with major negative public policy ramifications) can also lead to policy change.[17]

> ... every month we have that type of discussion, policy-making, more or less research-based, and then there are one or two cases that do not fit into that picture and are presented on television or on the front page of the newspapers and then the policy has to go two steps backward and start all over again.
>
> (health agency CEO)

Media events can also create 'policy windows' which offer a moment in time when there is a greater likelihood of positive policy change than would ordinarily be the case.[17] Research may be more effective at such times.

The writings of those directly engaged with developing best practice policy-making in government offer an account of complex, real world factors shaping policy and the use of evidence. For example, a publication on policy delivery from the Cabinet Office of the UK government emphasizes that

- policies are rarely fully formed when implemented: the ideal of policy being fully developed by evidence, which is very limited for specific policies, is unrealistic
- in decentralized government many individuals and dynamic systems will determine the meaning and delivery of policy
- policy can also be implemented in centralized command and control approaches that can include incremental change; in contrast, some policies are made and implemented at the 'grass roots' or community level and these can also have wide-ranging effects; other policies involve a mix of both of these
- to be effective much government policy involves changing behaviours and cultures, and research that fails to account for its assumptions about people is likely to lead to failed policies
- policies do not act singly but rather in an interdependent fashion with other policies.[18]

Key practical strategy

Models of how research may act to shape policy can be used by researchers to focus attention on particular aspects of this challenge. Such models are unlikely to offer an all-encompassing theory of what could happen in any one policy-making context.

Kinds and uses of information for policy

The diversity of information for policy

> . . . here in the UK we have the Dharzi policies. And in a couple of years Dharzi will be gone, there'll be another government and there will be a change in emphasis. You've got to use research that's very much focused on, say, public health, and the state of the nation, our changing population mix, the age profile—all of that material that's of very long standing—right through to the latest technological innovations that involve shared care between the specialist facility and the community practice in the home. So there's a great deal of material; what we've got to try and do is focus down on the elements that will help us with our business. Help us to understand why we should invest and dis-invest, where we should train and develop our workforce.
>
> (health agency CEO)

Studies of health policy decision-makers suggest that they use a broad variety of information: information about social and political beliefs and values, community consultations, expert opinion, statistical evidence, systematically collected and empirically validated evidence, observational studies, previous policies, legislation, protocols, anecdotal reports, popular internet sources, and so on.[19–21] Such studies problematize simplistic ideas about what is evidence for policy-making. Further, even within the different groups delivering research for and about health policy—economists, sociologists, political scientists, as well as health professionals of different kinds—there is considerable variation in what is meant by 'evidence'.[22]

The format of information is known to affect its use by policy-makers. For example, one study of state government policy-makers in the United States suggested that electronic information was used by younger officials in particular.[23] Another study of the uses of research-based information by decision-makers in Canadian community-based organizations suggested that they tended to use websites, research journals, electronic mail, conferences, and workshops.[24] The source of information can also shape its use: the United States-based study also suggested that organizations of government professionals were trusted sources of information for policy-makers.[23] However, such studies may be very context specific, with considerable variation in policy-makers' preferences, for example, for conference-based information.[24] One policy-maker advised the author:

> . . . you've got to try to scan the second grade research material that is done by masters degree students . . . there is a huge amount of students taking master degrees; they are presenting more or less elaborated material dealing with the local and national political processes that usually is not published any further . . . sometimes I find quite a lot of interesting trend material.
>
> (health agency CEO)

Not only are there different kinds, formats, and sources of information for policy, but also, as the previous section suggested, different levels and settings for policy-making will shape what configuration of evidence is used when. For example, study of the use of evidence in the development of some kinds of local health policies in the United Kingdom suggests that government reports and guidelines may be used to a greater extent than published research papers in these contexts, although internal experience also plays a major role.[25] At the international level, research into the use of evidence by the World Health Organization (WHO) suggests that it rarely uses systematic reviews and concise summaries of findings, but rather relies heavily on expert opinion.[26]

There is evidence also that the role or position that policy-makers have can influence the extent to which research is used. For example, public health programme managers and directors may use systematic reviews to a greater extent than some other policy-makers.[27] Different kinds of information may be more useful for different kinds of decisions. For example, studies of public health policy-making suggest that scholarly reviews can be more relevant to programme planning and justification, and have less influence on programme evaluation decisions.[25, 28]

It is also the case that information for health policy is brokered in different ways by different groups. There are views that government has become increasingly receptive to certain styles of evidence and that the number of stakeholder groups wanting to shape government opinion through the presentation of this evidence has increased in recent times.[21] Certainly, interest groups can have a controlling influence in presenting information that shapes government health policy, including in western democracies such as the United States where they form different kinds of permanent and temporary configurations. Their role is far more complex than it might have been in the 1960s and they are more numerous.[29]

> We have several what are called health care philanthropies and they're fairly well funded and they make grants to a lot of advocacy organisations and use really policy specific research to advance an advocacy agenda. So I think there's this interaction between what policy-makers develop an interest in and the health services research community here.
>
> (health agency CEO)

Another kind of interest group information brokering can be observed within the government itself. As the earlier point about state agencies suggested, health policy is also shaped by information coming from state and federal interactions and balances of power and interest groups operating within these interactions.[29]

Not enough is known about how senior health policy decision-makers understand sound decision-making, let alone evidence-based decision-making.[19] Nor is enough known about what kinds of research information (such as economic evaluation studies versus other kinds of evaluation studies) influence policy-making in what ways.[30] Even ostensibly practical kinds of evidence such as economic evaluation studies may not be used for a variety of reasons. These can range from lack of practical explanations of their relevance for policy-makers to policy-makers' inability to act on such evaluation results because of fiscal reasons.[30] Policy-makers may not be reliant on such apparently useful research because they combine information on cost-effectiveness with other kinds of information and values, and they operate with practical limitations created by, for example, constraints on healthcare resources.[31]

However, there is considerable support for the view that research evidence has a role, either before or after decision-making, selectively or more systematically, directly or indirectly.[19, 32, 33]

How research is utilized

Key practical strategy

An awareness of the different ways in which research might shape policy can be used by researchers in planning to maximize its usefulness. This may involve designing research to suit the desired way in which the evidence would be used by policy-makers. It may also involve planning to use different strategies such as personal contact with policy-makers to ensure the research is influential at the different levels of knowledge use by policy-makers.

> Once a policy-maker is interested in [a topic] I think the research is very influential in getting them on the right path to investing funds in interventions that are likely to be successful . . . I'm not sure that research often results in a policy-maker being interested in a topic. I know sometimes some of my health service researcher friends are frustrated because they feel they're working on something that's so very important . . .
>
> (health agency CEO)

A review by Hanney et al. of health research utilization concepts[4] suggests different ways in which research can shape policy:

1 through helping reconceptualize a policy problem

2 by providing empirical data for evidence-based decisions

3 by making explicit politically controlled opportunities or options, or the costs of not exercising particular options, which otherwise may not be so apparent

4 by providing a means for harnessing support from different interest groups

5 by offering a policy argument

6 by providing a new paradigm or framework for understanding policy realities

7 by developing the practice wisdom of policy-makers or their knowledge about what occurs at the health client-practitioner interface.[4]

The contemporary literature tends to emphasize the utilization of knowledge, including research, as occurring in stages, as part of a process, rather than simply in terms of outcomes. Thus knowledge and research utilization is conceptualized as a sequence of events that relates to different stages of the decision-making process.[34] Knott and Wildavsky describe seven stages of knowledge utilization which focus on what the policy-maker does:

1 reception: when the research evidence is actually received by the policy-maker

2 cognition: when the policy-maker has actually read and understood the research evidence

3 reference: when the evidence changes how the policy-maker understands the policy problem

4 effort: when the policy-maker makes an effort to apply the research evidence (regardless of the outcome; for example, even when political forces block the actual implementation of the research evidence)

5 adoption: when the research evidence actually influences the choice of policy options

6 implementation: when the research evidence actually shapes practice (not just policy)

7 impact: when the in-practice implementation of the research evidence actually delivers expected positive benefits (not just shapes policy or practice).[35]

In practice though, research is used in a manner that is far less tidy than such stages suggest. Research is used as part of a shifting and dynamic process—it's use is not limited to a single event or set of discrete and fixed linear stages.[36]

> I think some of the work coming out of the National Institute of Medicine around patient safety and health-care acquired infections has been influential in policy-making . . . but not sufficient to really get the policy agenda moving. It took groups that were more operational, I think, to get that agenda a really strong place in front of policy-makers . . . physician groups or patient safety groups who took the data and then told policy-makers why it mattered.
>
> (health agency CEO)

Research utilization can also be understood in terms of what actions happen in interactions and situations involving researchers and policy-makers, where the receptiveness of policy-makers and their contexts to evidence is important.[4] Maximizing the use of research is also about developing an awareness of multi-dimensional aspects of knowledge-making for policy—all the complex ways in which evidence can be made and can shape policy.[4]

The problem with 'evidence-based policy-making'

Policy decisions range quite significantly from very poorly made ones, loosely made ones, ad hoc, influenced by politics, reactionary, all the way across to strategically very well made, very well thought through, very well researched based, ones that you can have confidence in, ones that are outcome focused. There is the 'good zone' over there and the 'bad zone' over here, and then there's everything in between. I've seen them all and I've participated in them all: the good or the bad.

The ones that tend to be over to the left in my experience have tended to be poorer decisions and not necessarily cognisant of the system, of the needs out there, they're policy that's developed for want of expediency. But I've also seen some of the policy that's developed over on the right hand side to be a failure as well. And it's very interesting that it doesn't necessarily mean just because you've researched it well or you've got a good outcomes base that it's going to be the right policy for the environment you're in. So . . . it's not just about one component of what you're trying to look at. There is an awful lot of judgement, there's an awful lot of knowledge, historical knowledge that needs to be researched that you want to draw on, there is the expertise of community and people you want to draw on. So for me that all fits into that gammon, and it's a spectrum and it's never about one single thing.

(healthy agency CEO)

'Evidence-based policy-making' is a term used to describe an approach to policy-making that emphasizes that it be based on formal and systematically collected research evidence about what works and what does not work.[21] A focus on evidence does not mean one denies the reality that policy-making can often only be evidence-influenced or evidence-aware at best.[21] The discussion so far has emphasized the complexities of research-policy transfer. Studies of how policy-makers are using evidence in for instance, local NHS policy-making in the United Kingdom, suggest that research may be more likely to impact on policy in indirect ways. It may act indirectly to shape policy debate and the dialogue that takes place between service providers and users.[6] Another study of the impact of research on health equalities in the United Kingdom demonstrated that ideas, rather than research evidence, had become disseminated into health policy in three ways: successfully, partially, and in fractured ways.[37]

Such research suggests the value of having realistic expectations about the extent to which research can have a direct influence on policy, while ensuring that the many opportunities for it to shape policy, including indirectly, are known and exploited.[6] This is partly because, as complaints by policy-makers suggest, research evidence can rarely decisively establish causality. Rarely can it convincingly establish the attributions, connections, and exact relationships needed for really high stakes policy-making decisions.[38] In many cases there is not a large body of complete evidence linking treatment options to health status challenges that policy-makers could be using unproblematically in high stakes decision-making.[22]

The idea that research should be used as much as possible by policy-makers seems questionable in light of the possibility that well-informed policy may sometimes be possible when policy-makers do not rely on research. This may be so regardless of the apparent rigour of the research. As one observer has commented (not with reference to recent widening of the activities of the Cochrane Collaboration), 'The *Cochrane Library* is unlikely ever to contain systematic reviews or trials of the effects of redistributive national fiscal policies, or of economic investment leading to reductions in unemployment, on health'. Thus, issues like inequalities in health outcomes cannot be addressed effectively by a reliance on biomedical research, no matter how rigorous: from this perspective some argue that the Cochrane Collaboration has institutionalized a particular way of understanding what is evidence for policy.[39]

The fact that evidence-based policy has emerged from clinical medicine means that 'evidence-based policy' as we know it often involves an emphasis on randomized controlled trials (RCTs) that does not always recognize the contextualized needs of health policy-making.[40] This is because the policy decision-making context involves a shift from the individual-clinical level of evidence to systemic population and service development decision-making evidence.[34]

The possibility that evidence-based policy may not be well-informed policy is also suggested by the observations of Lavis et al. in the previously cited study of the uses of research by Canadian healthcare policy-makers. Lavis et al. wonder if future studies

> . . . might want to focus on the degree to which a policy was informed, not just on the extent to which the research is used. We were struck by our finding that for two cases in which research appears not to have been used, we considered the policymaking process particularly well informed. In both cases, structured processes gave play to a variety of research, other types of information, and values. Even more surprising to us, one of the cases in which research was used appeared to us to be one of the least informed policies. It seemed as if the effort to use as much research as possible for one policy issue (how much, 'in theory' to try to change) actually hindered a broader assessment of an equally important policy issue (what was not working before and why).[2] (p. 140)

Key ideas

In this book the argument is put forward that research practices can be developed in ways that help ensure policy is well-informed, not simply 'evidence-based'. This involves an engagement not only with generalizable truths, but also with local and particular policy problems and contexts.

> . . . evidence-based management is still quite in its infancy
>
> (health agency CEO)

What is policy-relevant research?

Key ideas

Recent literature has begun to make the distinction between analysis *of* policy and analysis *for* policy.[41] This distinction defines this book and its title. Analysis *of* policy offers an account of the nature and processes by which policy is made. Analysis *for* policy focuses on the needs of policy-makers and is a form of decision support.

> . . . we need a far better dialogue between researchers and policy-makers . . . this is a research system that's set up to reward people who write a more stock standard kind of research . . . And part of that's structural because we policy-makers don't control the research funding props.
>
> (health agency CEO)

Analysis for policy is a research effort that attempts to present evidence that influences policy. 'Analysis for policy' is thus a descriptive phrase that includes different kinds of research that act as textual interventions into policy practice.[42, 43] Analysis for policy has often concentrated on developing tools and forms of evidence that allow policy-makers to choose between different policy options.[41]

Policy-relevant research is a subset of analysis for policy. As the following chapters will suggest, policy-relevant research is research that has been developed more specifically as a set of practices for shaping policy. A review of health research defined one of the 'primary outputs' of research processes as journal articles, with outputs for policy-makers described as 'secondary outputs'.[4] In policy-relevant research, the primary research output is a policy solution or options crafted from a process of engagement with a specific policy problem. Often the sole, and always the main, aim of policy-relevant research is the production of these policy solutions. That aim may render it difficult to publish in scholarly journal publications without considerable reworking into a more scholarly genre.

The UK government's Cabinet Office publication *Professional Policy Making for the Twenty First Century* describes the desirable skills of policy-makers as including

- ◆ understanding the context—organizational, political, and wider—in which they are working
- ◆ managing complex relationships with a range of key players
- ◆ well-developed presentational skills, including the ability to work with others to gain ownership of their ideas by different groups
- ◆ a broader understanding of information technology and how it can be used to facilitate and support policy making
- ◆ a grounding in economics, statistics, and relevant scientific disciplines in order to act as 'intelligent customers' for complex policy evidence
- ◆ familiarity with using project management disciplines
- ◆ willingness to experiment, managing risks as they arise
- ◆ willingness to continue to learn new skills and acquire new knowledge throughout a career in policy making and elsewhere. (u.p.)[44]

The same report described the features of professional policy-making as policy-making that

- ◆ clearly defines outcomes and takes a long-term view, taking into account the likely effect and impact of the policy in the future 5 to 10 years and beyond
- ◆ takes full account of the national, European and international situation
- ◆ takes a holistic view looking beyond institutional boundaries to the government's strategic objectives
- ◆ is flexible and innovative, willing to question established ways of dealing with things and encourage new and creative ideas
- ◆ uses the best available evidence from a wide range of sources
- ◆ constantly reviews existing policy to ensure it is really dealing with problems it was designed to solve without having unintended detrimental effects elsewhere
- ◆ is fair to all people directly or indirectly affected by it and takes account of its impact more generally
- ◆ involves all key stakeholders at an early stage and throughout its development
- ◆ learns from experience of what works and what doesn't through systematic evaluation. (u.p)[44]

This book suggests that policy-relevant research is about helping policy-makers deliver this skill set and these features of good policy-making.

Health policy-making is known to have a distinctive knowledge base, culture, stakeholders, political influences, and so on.[41] Policy-relevant *health* research is a form of policy-relevant research that reflects how health policy operates with its own constraints and complexities distinguishing it from other areas such as education and welfare.[41]

Differences in the attributes of these different kinds of information—scholarly research about policy versus policy-relevant research—are more often a matter of degree than anything else. This book does not make black and white distinctions between the different forms of evidence and ways of shaping policy. It does suggest that much can be learned from separating out the more notable features of policy-relevant research for analysis and value-adding to the task of doing research for policy.

Barriers to research-policy transfer

. . . a lot of the esoteric research does seem to win the Brownie points, it does seem to get the accolades, but it never translates into anything on the ground which can bring about benefit and change and improvement . . . there's a lot of good basic science going on, but it's foremost to satisfy a closed community . . . it maybe does a great deal for a minority of people who can then use that to then get themselves appointments in other centres, both nationally and internationally.

(health agency CEO)

A list of barriers to research-policy transfer were given in the *British Medical Journal* by a UK commentator:

- Policymakers have goals other than clinical effectiveness (social, financial, strategic development of service, terms and conditions of employees, and electoral)
- Research evidence dismissed as irrelevant (from different sector or speciality, practice depends on tacit knowledge, not applicable locally)
- Lack of consensus about research evidence (complexity of evidence, scientific controversy, and different interpretations)
- Other types of competing evidence (personal experience, local information, eminent colleagues' opinions, and medico-legal reports)
- Social environment not conducive to policy change
- Poor quality of knowledge purveyors.[45]

Key ideas

Barriers to the use of research in policy-making are sometimes conceptualized as being of two types:

- barriers that are about the inherently complex nature of policy as a process that requires more than evidence: for example, factors to do with competing stakeholder group interests[22] and
- barriers that are about the fit between research evidence and policy-making needs: for example, when research evidence is not marshalled in a form, or sufficiency, that meets the contextual needs of policy-makers.[10, 22]

The first set of barriers suggest that perhaps research is, and even ought to be, one of only a range of ingredients in policy decision-making. Ideological, political, and/or strategic considerations may be more important to policy-makers than evidence. For example, the research literature suggests that (rightly or wrongly) the extent to which policy-makers view target populations as responsible for their health conditions may be an important influence on their willingness to allocate funds for programmes for those conditions and populations.[46] Conflicts between research and the current department values as expressed in philosophies, priorities, and strategies have been frequently cited as barriers to research-policy transfer—although research can present policy arguments that help ensure a better fit between the two.[47]

The two kinds of barriers reinforce the 'two worlds' hypothesis—that researchers and policy-makers occupy two different worlds and therefore the emphasis must be upon building bridges between the two worlds.[48] Such a view seems to reinforce the differences between researchers and policy-makers. For example, researchers may view policy-makers as motivated by political interests and power struggles rather than by the weight of empirical evidence and rational approaches to evidence-making. In contrast, policy-makers may see themselves as pragmatic and accountable to stakeholders, and view researchers as preoccupied with technicalities, jargon, and disconnected from 'real world' concerns.[49] The 'two worlds' hypothesis thus places strong emphasis on interaction and communication between the research and the policy-making worlds to overcome such differences.[49] This articulation between the two worlds involves a major commitment of resources and certain skills:

> . . . good research is happening here, there and everywhere but it is not always tied together . . . it takes a lot of commitment and resources to pull a series of research projects and outcomes together, distil them and then come up with policy directions . . . and that's not easy.

> (health agency CEO)

A review of studies using interview data from policy-makers themselves suggests that the 'two worlds' hypothesis may be true. It indicates that barriers most commonly reported were about the absence of personal interaction between policy-makers and researchers, poor timing of the research, irrelevance of the research, mutual mistrust, as well as power and budget struggles which may well be outside the control of the researcher.[49]

There are voices rejecting the 'two worlds' hypothesis as too simplistic. These voices have pointed out that the 'two worlds' hypothesis does not place enough onus on researchers to address the fundamental mismatch between the kind of evidence that they produce and that required for policy-making. From this perspective, the 'two worlds' hypothesis does not by itself help research to better account for the value-based dynamic, political, and contextual nature of policy-making.[48]

It is of course likely that the two kinds of barriers interact and therefore need to be addressed simultaneously by researchers for health policy. For example, economic and political considerations important to policy-makers can be taken into account when considering the form and kind of research they need.

What can and should researchers do to shape policy?

Literature suggests that there is much that the individual researchers can do to influence policy:

- *involving policy-makers in the research* through direct interaction with them, including through policy networks

- *timely relevance* and opportunistic use of 'policy windows' or key influencing events where researchers can translate their evidence

- *developing support for the research* through consensus-making in the community as well as by brokering the research evidence with key stakeholders

- *reviewing a wide range of evidence* to speak to the complex range of matters that define a policy problem

- *designing contextually sensitive research* that engages with the policy problem

- *triangulating and supplementing evidence* to ensure it is sufficient for the high stakes elements of policy decision-making

- *crafting a good policy argument* or 'policy story' from the empirical evidence that speaks persuasively to strategic and political concerns

- *crafting policy options sensitive to constraints* operating on policy-makers arising from legislative, policy, and procedural frameworks in which they operate

- *maximizing the effectiveness of implementation* by identifying enabling structures to help realize the policy options

- *maximizing the credibility and acceptability of results* through the involvement of policy-makers and community members in weighing the findings and policy options to be presented.[32, 49–52]

This book devotes much space to these ways of overcoming research-policy transfer.

Key ideas

The emerging consensus in literature is that an effective approach to research-policy transfer will involve a combination of strategies leading to interactive, multi-faceted knowledge transfer and exchange that builds relationships between researchers and research users, particularly policy-makers, on multiple levels.[24]

The independence of research

> I think we've had most success and the most satisfying relationships when we've talked to the research community early, where researchers have come and interviewed us about . . . their research question . . . and then they go back and think 'Well what kind of data are available, what kind of methods do we have to look at it to come up with a study?' Now we don't always agree that what they're measuring is exactly the right thing or that they are doing perfect work . . . but at least they're working on an issue that we've indicated the governor or the legislature is interested in solving.
>
> (health agency CEO)

Each of the ways of overcoming barriers to research-policy transfer brings their own challenges. However, the exhortation that decision-makers be involved in almost every stage of the research to help bring a focus to their needs, assisting its use and take-up, can be particularly challenging. On the one hand it is argued that this involvement need not necessarily compromise the independence of the research—that it can bring a strong contextual validity to the research, enhancing its quality.[53] On the other hand, the challenges of ensuring that research evidence does not suffer from political interference can be considerable. A significant body of literature has developed to suggest that researchers in many different settings are subjected to efforts to politicize or silence objective scientific research, efforts that grow increasingly more sophisticated.[54] Even, and perhaps especially, randomized controlled studies for policy have been subjected to political interference in ways that affect their rigour and validity.[55] Ways in which this interference operates may include

- economic manipulation (where the researcher is economically indebted to the policy-maker)
- delaying tactics to help ensure the policy opportunity or window has passed
- attacking the value of research

◆ falsely presenting counter-research or arguments; for example, when vested economic interests masquerade as grassroots community organizations or as research organizations

◆ harassment of researchers; for example, by suing them.[54]

The nature of this challenge will be shaped by the power dynamic operating in the research setting. Academics in university institutional settings will face quite different challenges from those who work within policy research units in government or as independent consultants. However, it is important to keep in mind that the integrity of policy contexts is as diverse as their nature. There are policy-makers who have very little to gain from trying to suppress, distort, or otherwise manipulate research. Their political survival in democratic systems may rely on the capacity of research to provide effective translation of community preferences and policy feasibility.

This is not to obscure the reality, as leading United States commentator Wildavsky has argued in his 1987 monograph, *Speaking Truth to Power*, that warring elites or 'interest group politics' shape much of what happens in public policy.[7] The emphasis on political accounts of health policy-making is important in many health policy histories.[29] It suggests that sometimes the values are non-negotiable. The scholarly policy research also contains accounts that assert how policy-makers define the problem can be a part of the problem. Therefore, accepting the research brief can mean accepting definitions that can ideologically compromise the researcher: [56]

> There's an awful lot of research questions that come from 'Justify this for me' or 'Construct it in a way to support the decision that the policy-makers want to make, are going to make'. I think that's bad research because it doesn't actually help you inform policy. And it's probably motivated by some managerial, political or ad hoc approach to research. But I want researchers who sit down and say 'How should you design a perfect health care delivery system?' and research around what policy you need to implement that, around the social fabric of society, around the cultural influences, around how much you've got to spend, what the disease profiles are. You know that's where you would really love to be, doing that and asking 'So what would be the most interesting, the most beneficial policy for achieving that?'
>
> (healthy agency CEO)

However, it is hard to believe that the values of policy decision-makers cannot be mediated by research. Public sector researchers always have some degree of choice about what values they serve, to what extent; particularly since the intellectual arts are sufficiently abstruse that there is room for forms of resistance through reinterpretation, including as part of community consensus-making. Such possibilities for resistance are identified, theorized, and modelled throughout this book. Wildavsky's 1987 monograph, with its emphasis on the politicization of public policy analysis and the importance of understanding human relations and social practices in the formation of public policy, offers a basis for reflecting on what research can do as a form of social practice to shape and influence those human relations.[7] This emphasis on quality social practices to mediate and reinforce desirable social values, as much as written and analytic techniques, lies at the heart of policy-relevant research.

Thus, the idea that researchers can maintain their integrity as providers of policy-relevant evidence, not political spin, need not position them in a passive role as transmitters of that evidence. For example, and as Chapter 6 on consensus-making suggests, researchers can also influence policy-making by actively building the capacity of community members to speak collectively to policy-makers.

Key ideas

Policy-relevant research is a genre that gives researchers an active role in achieving policy change. In this genre researchers do much more than simply reproduce the policy-maker's values: they seek to illuminate, reinterpret, and even shape the policy-maker's views and actions through written as well as social practices.

Can policy-relevant solutions be delivered on time?

. . . good innovative centres see the horizons coming. They network clinically, internationally. They observe research that's beginning to emerge, even when some of it is a little tenuous and crude, and build upon that and then work towards appropriate change. It does tend to take a government some time to take all of that on board, to be able to have the confidence to publish and endorse good practice and promote change or investment.

There's quite a timing issue; there's always a timeline. That's understandable, so I think when you're in a large clinical centre the role really is to keep pushing the boundaries, to continue innovating and not always wait for the well-founded evidence-based practice.

(health agency CEO)

We need more mechanisms for . . . you might say 'quick and juicy research.'

(health agency CEO)

As this chapter has suggested, researchers can do much to overcome barriers to the use of evidence by policy-makers. Yet there is no doubt that one of the more challenging of these barriers is the crisis-oriented nature of policy-making which may not always permit timely delivery of evidence.[57]

However, claims that research can only *very rarely* shape policy because there is no time in policy-making for a solution to be researched and tested, should be viewed critically. The complexities of the 'real life' evidence examined in this book at least suggest that they simplify what actually happens. Such claims sometimes belong to enlightenment models of research and may come from a 'batten down the hatches' approach to scholarly research, defending the methodological status quo. They do not seem to admit the possibility that researchers should and can adapt to the needs of policy-makers.

Claims that evidence cannot be used to deliver solutions for policy-makers because 'all is flux' in policy-making contexts also fail to account for the ways in which policy contexts and problems have similarities across time. Different language can be used by different policy-makers over time to describe the same policy problem. Further, as Wildavsky has observed, 'more and more public policy is about coping with consequences of past policies'[7] (p. 4). This includes coping with the effects of the 'policy pendulum' which swings back and forth from the values of the political right to those of the left:

> The broader lesson from Singapore is that health care reform continues to swing back and forth between a belief in market forces and the use of government regulation. In reality, health policy is replete with examples of market failures and government failures as policy makers experiment with different instruments. The variety of health care systems developed around the world indicates that the choice is neither pure markets nor government control but the balance to be struck between the two.[58] (p. 744)

Policy-relevant research is about engaging with such continuities in policy-making, as much as with what is different about the moment. It is a fact sometimes forgotten by scholarly researchers outside public policy-making contexts that many researchers in those policy contexts know that policy past intimately precisely because they inhabited it. This is part of the reason researchers working in public policy contexts can sometimes move with greater speed to identify and respond to particular policy contexts.

Key ideas

The barriers to delivering policy solutions using research are not simply about the future arriving too quickly to be prepared. As further explained in Chapter 3 on practices of reviewing, in policy-relevant research it is also critical to speedily decipher the legacies of the past.

Key recommended reading

Nutley S, Walter I, Davies H. *Using Evidence: How Research can Inform Public Services.*
Bristol, The Policy Press, 2007.

Case studies in what changes health policy

Case study: The Acheson report—tackling inequalities of health in the United Kingdom

A UK health policy report published in 1998 by Professor Donald Acheson—the *Independent Inquiry into Inequalities in Health*[59]—offers one example of the complex art of 'getting it right' for health policy-makers. The aim of this report was to undertake a government review summarizing the evidence of inequalities of health and life expectancy in England and identify evidence-based policy for reducing health inequalities. That aim was shaped by the strategic policy-making needs of the new Blair government at a particular historical moment. Britain had experienced 18 years of Conservative rule which had brought prosperity at the price of growing inequality and social division. This created powerful impetus for new directions in public policy towards greater equality[60]—a 'policy window' not present 20 years before when a similar report[61] was presented to the British government.

The focus in the Acheson report on health inequalities linked to complex structural inequalities in British society meant that it had to draw on a wide range of evidence beyond classical experimental designs. Concluding that 'controlled intervention studies are rare' the report explains that

> Indeed, the more a potential intervention relates to the wider determinants of inequalities in health (i.e. 'upstream' policies), the less the possibility of using the methodology of a controlled trial to evaluate it. We have, therefore, evaluated many different types of evidence in forming our judgement.[59]

Thus, the inquiry had to proceed in a context where there was little hard empirical evidence of 'what works'. Much of the available evidence did not offer proposals focusing on relevant changes to legislation and policy.[62] The community among which Acheson sought consensus was primarily the community of experts across multiple disciplines who could help synthesize evidence about the diverse structural determinants of health inequality. The inquiry received a wide range of submissions from the community and commissioned papers from experts on 17 topics such as income, housing, and transport. The policy argument that the report presented drew on arguments to do with equity and social efficiency based on a socioeconomic model of the causes of health inequalities. These were used to support recommendations for change to a wide range of areas, from education to housing to transport that went far beyond recommendations to do with healthy behaviours. The Acheson report had arguable success—the holistic outcomes of its inter-governmental recommendations were difficult to measure. Yet there can be no doubt it helped put health inequalities at the centre of the British government's efforts to produce a healthier nation.[63] As such it offers an example of not only the complexities of a particular genre of policy-relevant evidence, but also the importance of context and political will in ensuring that research is used.

Case study: Chronic care reform (diabetes) in the United State's private healthcare sector

The United States has a decentralized healthcare system in which the federal government sets policy for Medicare, state and local governments develop policies for the areas where they have responsibility, and the private sector also makes policy decisions. In such a context, what changes health policy?

This case study deals with how research informed policy in the case of one private agency, Kaiser Permanente, drawing on the published account of this work by Steifel and others.[64]

The challenge was how to ensure the scientific and clinical research about chronic conditions informed healthcare, in this example diabetes. The award-winning Integrated Diabetes Care (IDC) Programme was the first of a portfolio of care management programmes developed by the Kaiser Permanente's Care Management Institute (CMI). The role of CMI was to bridge the gap between research and policy. The steps involved were:

♦ Translation of clinical research into a rationale for care management programmes for priority populations by the CMI

♦ Priority-setting by Kaiser Permanente policy-makers to decide the sub-populations to target

♦ The care management programme was developed by CMI staff working with clinical and operational experts

♦ The resulting care management programme was reviewed and approved by Kaiser Permanente policy decision-makers

♦ The CMI staff worked with a network of regional staff to implement the programme

♦ CMI staff developed and coordinated a performance measurement system using a network of clinical and operational staff

♦ CMI staff supported the ongoing implementation of the chronic care management programme

♦ There was an ongoing cycle of performance measurement and policy development coordinated by CMI staff, which provided continuous review of the programme.

The research methods used were designed to meet policy-making needs. For example, programmes were evaluated using 'Archimedes', a biomathematical simulation model developed by Kaiser Permanente that models both disease and care processes. It simulates the progression of diabetes as well as its complications in a population, allowing for estimations of the impact of different kinds of care management approaches over time. The information produced by the model offered a basis for policy decision-making about which care management approaches were effective.

The approach saw dramatic improvements in diabetes care and management outcomes among members of the Kaiser Permanente. It was characterized by a process of policy change that was iterative, managed by a translational policy research unit acting as a conduit between policy-makers, clinical researchers, operational and clinical experts. This case study also highlights that, at different stages of the policy development process, different kinds of research can be used to influence different kinds of policy decisions. For example, research giving the rationale for changing approaches to particular sub-populations was used to consider priority-setting for those sub-populations.

This example also highlights that policy development in the health sector is largely about achieving a complex goal at the patient level: changed health outcomes. To achieve that goal, clinicians and operational managers identified in the regions were co-opted to serve on working groups, as well as other aspects of development of the initiative. CMI staff also worked closely with clinicians to design implementation of the policy around the way they worked in order to help ensure success of the policy.

Chapter 2

Deciphering the policy problem

The task of deciphering the policy problem

Overview

Deciphering the policy problem is a critical challenge in the preparatory work required to deliver policy-relevant research. The extent to which the evidence delivers workable solutions for clearly understood policy problems is a critical measure of the success of research for policy-makers. An accurate reading of the policy problems is a critical task in policy-relevant research because this reading will be used to drive the design of the whole research enterprise. This chapter aims to help the researcher with that task.

> . . . it's absolutely right that sometimes what you think is the problem isn't actually the problem.
>
> (health agency CEO)

> . . . we're not doing enough research in the areas of the true directions of the health care. We seem to be doing research around the periphery rather than trying to answer the real fundamental questions. Once you get to grips with that you can get many more of the questions that you need: about how do you get quality in the way you deliver care for people, how do you get lower hour rates, how do you get efficient effective management of resources, how do you get the right employment and workforce around it?
>
> (health agency CEO)

As noted in Chapter 1, some views of policy-making suggest that policy problems are so amorphous that they cannot be deciphered and responded to in a timely fashion. Chapter 1 also highlighted the view that scholars may have trouble engaging with policy problems because such problems are ideologically defined. There are elements of truth to all this, just as there is some truth in the argument that traditional methods of scholarship poorly equip researchers to meet the demands of deciphering and redefining the policy problem.

Policy problems present a challenge because they are rarely given in a neatly wrapped package. Nor can the researcher formulate them using a literature review, no matter how exhaustive. Rather, the researcher must read the policy problems from a variety of carefully assembled written and unwritten information. The policy problem is a creature of a particular context and must be effectively redefined if the researcher is to offer research that helps policy-makers. The definition of the policy problem is also a site of political struggle. Deciphering the policy problem is also about redefining policy-makers' understandings of it in ways that are ultimately useful:

> . . . what is useful is to be able to come up with slightly different hypotheses . . . encourage policy-makers to look at things differently, to try novel approaches and policy innovation.
>
> (health agency CEO)

The task of deciphering the policy problem can be approached systematically. It involves several key elements:

- managing the policy briefing
- assembling policy and other key documents and reading their sub-texts in politically sensitive contexts where the language used to describe the policy challenge may be misleading
- establishing informal networks useful to triangulating the researchers' reading of the policy problem
- using those close to policy decision-makers to help audit the researcher's developing understanding of the policy problem
- interpreting the policy problems in ways that allow the researcher to manage and engage productively with ideology

The importance of context in deciphering the policy problem

> I think it's very important to try to follow from day to day more or less, or at least from month to month, the running issues in the specific field, trying to scan political documents, legislative preparations, supervisory reports, administrative documents, the media . . . Trying to have some kind of an intelligence of it, scanning the environment, scanning the political debate . . . because then you can see what are the possible questions that should be answered by research, what are the words that are used, what are the valid concepts, what is the current value basis for the political work . . . some kind of intelligence service, if you could call it that, should be set up by researchers trying to follow specific health policy fields.
>
> (health agency CEO)

Policy-relevant research is, from beginning to end, shaped by an interpretation of a local and particular policy challenge, distilled into a policy problem, and the need to find policy solutions for this problem (or problems). The word 'local' is not used here in any simple geographical sense; it refers to the idea that there are specific loci or sites (global, national, regional, civic etc.) relevant to understanding the challenges and problems that shape policy-making. Thus, global policy-making in health has its own loci or contexts.

Key ideas

Context is a mix of distinctive policy objectives, how effects are modified, resources are constrained, and community and political interests operate in a particular policy decision-making situation. It refers to the whole complex of historical, cultural and socio-political forces that shape the distinctiveness of any one policy environment.[65]

This book emphasizes the importance of context for policy-makers who often feel that researchers do not understand the structures and constraints within which they work, thus preventing much research transfer into policy.[52, 66, 67] It is not enough that research for policy be of good scientific merit.[68, 69] It is known that research that leaves out the profoundly contextual problem-solving required ('what will work for this particular place') results in ill-informed policies.[2] A focus on policy decision-makers' needs and contexts is positively associated with research take-up.[69]

> ...you have to first of all understand everything you can possibly understand about the political side of things, the financial side of things, the community side of things, and take all of that into consideration when you formulate your research project.
>
> (health agency CEO)

Explicit, implicit, and pragmatic dimensions of policy-maker's needs and context

> 'I think being very clear and being focused about understanding the policy and game is critical, because that helps to set the boundaries and areas in which you don't go into because you know that will be a non-starter as far as policies are concerned ... having a mind to what is implementable, what is pragmatic, what is a reasonable way forward, would also help.
>
> (health agency CEO)

Chapter 1 defined the policy problem as being comprised of the tensions, barriers, and challenges associated with a particular policy goal and context. The policy problem also requires the researcher to 'read' the implicit, explicit, and pragmatic needs and context of the policy-maker bound up in the policy goals.

The implicit needs could be different from the stated needs which in turn could be different from what is pragmatically possible for the policy-maker. The policy problem should be read in a way that accounts for these three things. For example, the researcher may be

- implicitly asked to find out whether an intervention will be acceptable to a particular group
- explicitly asked to find out what works for whom in which circumstances

but

- pragmatically in the interests of feasible policy-making may need to focus the research effort on acceptability for three key stakeholder groups.

Majone distinguishes the stable or critical elements of a policy context from those elements that lie on the periphery and can be changed.[16] Both of these kinds of elements need to be deciphered. Both may be explicit or implicit. Both may never have been perceived or consciously articulated by the policy-makers themselves. This is what makes the task of deciphering the policy problem an art that includes not just data gathering and networking but also reflection, theorising, and hypothesising.

Key practical strategy

There is no easy answer to the question of how to decipher the implicit dimensions of the policy problem. Researchers should pay attention to gaps and silences in policy documents, as well as observe different groups of stakeholders *in situ*, such as clients, service providers, and policy-makers themselves.[70] The task of deciphering the policy problem is essentially an iterative task that will take place over the entire course of the research effort for policy-making.

Many of the research methods explored in this book aim to capture the contextual richness important to perceiving the implicit dimensions of the policy problem.

Constraints on policy-makers

Part of the task of deciphering the policy problem is also about deciphering constraints which may be implicit or explicit; whether they are about values and contextual political factors, history, culture, or budget constraints.[31] For example, different kinds of budget constraints operate in different ways to shape the policy challenge. In health there are constraints on partial budgets for successive periods or for specific conditions of patient groups. These may be operating in different permutations and ways to shape the policy decisions that are possible.[31] Majone describes constraints on policy-makers as a complex web of limitations;

> [. . .] prior policies and institutional inertia; inadequate, outdated, or wrong information; cognitive limitations; the plans of other policymakers and the resistance of one's own bureaucracy; vested interests and the demands and aspirations of different social groups; limits on the span of control and on the available time and resources; authority leakage and loss of legitimacy; foreign commitments and international pressures.[71] (p. 75)

As Majone explains, constraints may also be self-imposed. The range of such self-imposed constraints may be adopted for a limited purpose or time (like contractual commitments); accepted 'until further notice' (particular administrative regulations); critical to the achievement of certain policy goals (deference to other policy-makers or stakeholders); constraints that are accepted implicitly (like cultural norms).[16]

A meaningless interpretation of a policy problem will deliver policy options that cannot work because they do not account for such constraints. Thus, even in economic evaluations, assuming that simply producing a set of cost-effectiveness ratios is enough to resolve the policy problem is probably a mistake.[31] So is searching for theories or data that will deliver up a universal statement of the policy challenge.[31] The challenge is about engaging with such contextual constraints in ways that bring local as well as generic or broader knowledge and skills together.

Deciphering trade-offs

Deciphering policy 'trade-offs' is an important part of the task of deciphering the health policy problem. Policy goals are often not singular. They may be comprised of multiple related or even inconsistent objectives. Realistically, it will be difficult to find policy options that can simultaneously achieve all aspects of the policy goal. A 'trade-off' is an element of a policy goal the policy-maker is willing to sacrifice to some degree in the interests of achieving another element of the goal. Research for policy-making needs to be informed by information about the kinds of trade-offs that policy decision-makers are willing to make between such things as equity, quality, safety, cost, efficiency, and so on in a particular context.[20] Such research often needs to model the possible trade-offs that can be made between these different elements of a policy goal.

The task of deciphering the policy problem includes knowing the difference between a policy goal and a policy constraint. As Majone explains, an objective constraint outside the control of the policy-maker cannot be so easily traded off against other constraints or goals. Many self-imposed constraints also cannot be so easily traded-off. Thus, elements of policy goals can often be traded off, whereas many constraints cannot be traded off.[16]

Trade-offs are not simply about what the policy-makers are willing to sacrifice. They are also about the difference between what policy-makers imagine might work and what the available information suggests is possible. Policy-relevant research can offer valuable information about what implementing one aspect of a policy goal will mean for achieving other aspects of a policy goal. For example, locating a hospital in the rural north of a state may achieve political results in that community, but at the cost of safety and quality because of the history of problems attracting specialists to that area.

Accordingly, in an imperfect world, with multiple competing objectives and interests, policy-makers often need to be given evidence that identifies and models the trade-offs they will need to make to achieve—usually only partially—their policy goals. Policy-relevant research can have added value to policy-makers when it synthesizes the evidence about such trade-offs in ways that are accessible not simply to policy-makers, but also community members to whom policy-makers must explain such trade-offs.

The policy-problem: deciphering uncertainty and the problem of innovation

> Not only in my experience does the research come too late; it is more retrospective and looking backwards than actually informing policy going forwards.
>
> (health agency CEO)

The policy problem is also about deciphering what must be resolved in the light of what is uncertain. In practice this does not represent a discrete preliminary stage of the research for policy-makers. Rather, it is ongoing throughout the review and formal data collection exercises. This chapter deals more with what needs to be done at the outset to obtain preliminary understandings of the policy problem. Researchers who identify what is unknown at the *end* of the process of research can also help policy-makers understand the true nature of the policy problem and its best solution. The dynamic nature of policy contexts means that the policy option will almost inevitably be a decision taken about the future in a context of uncertainty. This means that research for policy is also to some extent about helping policy-makers manage uncertainty.

The management of risk by policy-makers presents them with a very considerable challenge: change brings risk, but so does not changing. Risk management is a complex area of health policy operation that can bring with it a highly structured approach to identifying, assessing, and controlling risks, with well-defined steps. Some research for policy can be strongly focussed on helping policy-makers meet the challenges of risk management: identifying mechanisms that can help minimize risk, designing processes that help monitor risks and control them if they materialize, as well as offering frameworks for decision-making about risk.[72]

Risk-taking is thus an almost inevitable element of the policy context. Risk may not be resolved because, as the UK Cabinet Office publication *Professional Policy Making for the Twenty First Century* states, 'Being innovative usually involves taking risks and effective policy making must encompass the identification, assessment and management of risk. (u.p.)[44] This report went on to conclude from its review of policy-making practices in the UK that risks were not being identified 'let alone actively managed':

> ... we found a widespread view that civil service culture does not welcome new thinking or change. Outsiders tend to perceive policy makers as inward looking. There is general acceptance that fear of failure and the high penalties attached to 'mistakes' are powerful disincentives to real innovation. Policy makers often do not choose to take risks, in part, because of the way Parliament and other external bodies hold them to account, but also because there is a belief that career progression depends more on being 'a safe pair of hands' than on being innovative. (u.p.)[44]

This situation of uncertainty and the demands of risk management is thus part of the task of deciphering the policy problem. The critical elements of the policy problem include managing uncertainty in relation to three key areas: how viable the options are, how manageable the risks are, and whether the benefits can be realized in practice.[72] These are questions that literature review and the processes of data collection also need to address.

A tool for deciphering policy problems

The foregoing discussion suggests that policy problems are about deciphering a whole range of uncertainties and constraints, and the trade-offs that may be possible. To do this effectively, the researcher will need to identify what is known and what is not known about the policy problem. A useful conceptual paper on the subject of uncertainty in both a technical-mathematical and policy-making sense is provided by Walker et al. [1] It invites the researcher to reflect on the nature of the uncertainty, what the level of uncertainty is, and the source or cause of the uncertainty.[1] One of the strengths of this approach for policy-relevant research is that it recognizes that the uncertainty of research methods is part and parcel of the uncertainty of the dynamics of a policy context. Table 2.1 offers a simplified and adapted (for health policy purposes) version of the table offered by Walker and colleagues.

Table 2.1 Table of uncertainty—a tool for deciphering policy problems

Kind of certainty or uncertainty	Definition: describe the nature of the certainty or uncertainty	Level: describe the level of the uncertainty or certainty e.g. level of statistical uncertainty, levels of scenario uncertainty under different options, and of recognized ignorance etc.	Source: describe the source of the uncertainty or certainty, e.g. different kinds of imperfections in the knowledge base etc.
Certainty in the policy context: bio-medical, technological, social, political etc. certainties			
Uncertainty in the policy context: bio-medical, technological, social, political etc. uncertainties			
Certainty in the research model: certainties to do with the conceptual and technical research models to be used to deliver policy options etc.			
Uncertainty in the research model: uncertainties to do with the conceptual and technical research models to be used to deliver policy options etc.			
Certainty in the inputs for what is known: influences on policy-makers, data about the system etc.			
Uncertainty in the inputs for what is known: influences on policy-makers, data about the system etc.			
Certainty in the outcomes of different actions: certainty about end results			
Uncertainty in the outcomes of different actions: uncertainty about end results			

The columns and rows can of course, be further divided—the specificity of every policy context means that any such table in a book such as this can offer only a conceptual point of departure for mapping what is known and what is not known about a particular policy problem. New categories will need to be developed to suit the context. This table can also be adapted to suit the number of policy options that may need to be differentiated as these develop. Ideally, the categories used in the table will be developed in dialogue between researchers and policy decision-makers, as well as community stakeholders.

The table should also be developed with reference to scholarly literature. For example, there are theoretical models of resource allocation, including resource constraints, which can offer useful ways of conceptualizing what is known about resource constraints in a particular health policy setting. The better ones have been developed with the input of policy-makers to describe what happens in practice.[31] However, care needs to be taken to ensure that such theoretical models do not 'blinker' the researcher to the importance of developing a table that is tailored to the needs of the specific context. Useful discussion of the nature of uncertainty in communicating data to the broader community is given the 2009 book *Making Data Talk: The Science and Practice of Translating Public Health Research and Surveillance Findings to Policy Makers, the Public, and the Press by* Nelson, Hess, and Croyle.[73]

The table can be used to drive the design, and incorporate the results of, each stage of the research, such as the literature review and data collection in the community. However, it is not proposed that such a table be copied into the final report to policy-makers. Rather, such tables are probably best used as tools to guide the researcher's thinking, to ensure that the challenges of responding to particular uncertainties are not simplified or lost along the way. Tables such as these can be helpful precisely because not all areas of uncertainty will be known in the preliminary stages of deciphering the policy problem. Accordingly, the table should be seen as a continually evolving device for research planning and implementation, at the literature review, data collection, analysis, and policy options development stages—as previously unknown uncertainties emerge, or are resolved, and what appeared certain once no longer seems so.

The different components of the policy problem

A recent book by Knoepfel *Public Policy Analysis* highlights the different types of public policy analysis needed for solving the different elements of the policy problem, simplified here as analyses of

+ social and political definitions of the policy problem and its causes, which are themselves the product of struggle between different competing groups
+ the political-administrative programmes and arrangements at stake for solving the policy problem, including legislative and regulatory decisions that must be made, as well as competencies, responsibilities, and resources available

- action plans and outputs needed for solving the policy problem, including priorities for implementation in the context of geography, society, and time considerations, and related actions
- impacts and results of actions for target groups relevant to the policy problem and understanding the efficacy of policy solutions.[74]

This list can be used by researchers to audit their understandings of the policy problem.

Key practical strategy

As the project progresses, researchers may wish to add to the table of uncertainty given in this chapter in the light of their consideration of the different kinds of policy analyses needed for different components of the policy problem. These different kinds of analyses addressing the different parts of the policy problem will also need to be informed by what is known and what is not known. Thus the detail of the different research analyses needed can be added to the description of certainty and uncertainty for 'the research model' in the table of uncertainty. Thinking about different kinds of policy analyses that might be needed for different parts of the policy problem can help clarify the nature of the policy problem.

Recommended reading

Walker W, Harremoes P, Rotmans J, et al. Defining uncertainty: A conceptual basis for uncertainty management in model-based decision support. *Integrated Assessment* 2003; 4(1): 5–17.

The chapters that follow offer ways of doing the different kinds of policy analyses that may be needed.

Case studies in deciphering the policy problem

Case study in deciphering the policy problem: Making health choices easier in the UK

The 2004 National Health Service (NHS) report *Choosing Health: Making Healthy Choices Easier*[75] offers an example of how a complex policy problem was represented. The issue of people managing their own health in ways that promote good health outcomes lies at the centre of the report. In a modern democratic system this represents a considerable policy challenge: on the one hand, there are arguments that the UK government needed to do more to limit individual choices leading to unhealthy outcomes and, on the other, that such choices should be restrained only by the forces of the free market. How was this policy challenge interpreted in the report?

The interpretation of the policy problem was made more complex because the meaning of 'choice' is shaped by politics. Choice is described in this report as being influenced by socio-economic circumstances and other forms of disadvantage that make it easier for some to exercise options for healthier lifestyles. The report explains that, from the perspective of the UK Labour government, choice is limited for some and thus it is the government's role to make the playing field more level for all. For the Labour government the policy problem becomes ostensibly about how to give all citizens *equal opportunity* to make healthy life choices. At the same time, the report suggests that the UK government faces the parallel challenge of also ensuring that the free exercise of choice does not infringe on the rights of others. This includes the rights of children to a healthy life.

Such a policy challenge is very complex and will require long-term, inter-systemic approaches based on carefully developed, evidence-based understandings of the component parts of the policy problem.

The report uses a body of research to develop and nuance the definition of the policy problem. It suggests the explicit, implicit, and pragmatic dimensions of policy-makers' needs, their constraints, possible trade-offs, and areas of ongoing uncertainty.

For example, the population health data used in the report suggest that despite great gains in health generally in England over the last century, inequalities in health have persisted. The report notes that some parts of England today have the same mortality rates as the national average in the 1950s. It also shows that new kinds of inequalities have emerged. One of these is mental health: not only has there been an increase in mental health problems, but mental health conditions are more common in areas of socio-economic deprivation. Discussion of these new and continuing health policy challenges is supported in the report with evidence from a wide range of sources: recent policy initiatives, national and international data, as well as the results of the consultations conducted for the report.

The extensive consultations undertaken—over 150,000 individuals were involved—clarified the constraints on government intervention, further nuancing the policy problem as it could be understood. It suggested that there was no strong community support for government involvement in a wide range of private health choices. The community wanted the role of government to be about providing information and practical support for healthy choices. However, there was support for government to act in areas where an individual's choices affected the rights of another to have a healthy life, and where government could have a strong role in social justice by addressing the underlying social causes of ill-health. Through these consultations the policy challenge was defined as being about how to make healthy choices easier for people within a framework that protected their rights and fostered equal opportunity to become healthy.

The general policy challenge 'How to make healthy choices easier for people within a framework that protects their rights and fosters equal opportunity to become healthy' is too broad to be useable. To be in a form that researchers can use to marshal evidence and solutions, and policy-makers can use to make practical decisions, the policy problem needs to be translated into its constituent parts. Each of the parts of the policy problem can then be addressed with a view to what works. In the report *Choosing Health: Making Healthy Choices Easier* the general policy problem was further explored in its larger and smaller parts, which for the sake of analysis can be conceptualized here as 'macro' policy problems (big parts of the general policy problem) and their 'micro' policy aspects (smaller constituent parts of the macro policy problem).

For example, in the report, one macro aspect of the general policy problem relates to the question 'How do you create demand for healthy choices in a market economy?' This was elaborated through, for example, discussion of health marketing, in specific health areas such as sexual health, obesity, and smoking, for different social groups such as ethnic minorities and disadvantaged groups. In this way, discussion of the constituent parts of the macro-policy challenge could be broken down into useable micro-policy statements of the policy problem. One such micro-policy challenge was: how do you get good information about healthy choices relevant to diabetes to a largely Asian community that is often living in economically stressed circumstances, with limited English language access, and with distinctive shopping and television watching preferences?

A further example of a macro challenge is represented in the report in the form of the question 'How can children be protected and nurtured to develop healthy choices as part of a whole-of-community approach?' Meeting such macro-policy changes in this report involves looking across a wide range of challenges (all children, all parents, and services) to support development of healthy framework for life. Consideration of different aspects of this framework could then lead to consideration of different kinds of solutions at the micro-level. For example, the report considers the challenge of under-age smoking, including how to counteract the problem of under-age smoking. It refines the understanding of the policy problem by considering evidence that existing initiatives have not stopped the problem from being a major policy concern. It further diagnoses the policy problem by demonstrating with reference to evidence that, for example, most children who try to buy cigarettes from retail outlets find it relatively easy to do so.

Discussion of solutions to these micro policy problems is developed in the report, in relation to key principles, government targets and existing policy, information about service contexts and service capabilities, local and national case study experience, tools and models, and the available research evidence.

Thus, by translating the general policy problem from the macro to the micro level, a seemingly insurmountable general policy challenge is understood in ways that lead to specific actionable policy solutions or decision-points.

Case study: Defining the policy problem of health workforce in rural and regional Australia

In 2008 the Australian government released its *Report on the Audit of Health Workforce in Rural and Regional Australia* which provided an audit of the shortage of doctors, nurses, and other allied health professionals in these areas.[76] Its main value is as an elaboration of the nature of the policy problem through detailed discussion of the nature and reasons for such shortages. The report was expected to inform policy understandings in the Rudd government which was swept into power in 2007 on election promises that included commitments to improve services to rural and regional Australia. The need for clearer policy understandings of this complex challenge was seen as critical in a context in which the previous Australian government had conducted, but not released, studies on this controversial subject.

The method used was compilation and analysis of recent workforce data from multiple sources, community submissions and informal input from around 40 key stakeholders, as well as a literature review. First, the report explores the distribution of the health workforce in rural and regional Australia, presenting issues to do with the quality and coverage of available data. It offers information on workforce supply, including information about numbers and proportions of Australian and overseas-trained health professionals in the rural and regional workforce. Information about population trends that will have an impact on health needs is also included. Second, stakeholder input is presented in ways that triangulate and supplement the picture that emerges from these data. Third, the report includes a review of the scholarly and applied literature on the roles of health professionals, nationally and internationally. These sources are synthesized into key findings that aim to develop policy understandings of the nature of the policy problem.

The report provided findings which suggested that the supply of doctors was low to very poor, and the supply of other health professionals was low to poor, in many rural and regional areas of Australia. However, the supply of nurses was found to be relatively even across Australia. It found that supply and distribution corresponded with the distribution of state and territory funded health services across Australia. The report found that modest increases in the medical workforce in rural and remote Australia had not kept pace with population growth, and had been achieved by restricting areas where overseas doctors can practice. It suggested that access to services was not simply about the distribution of workforce, but also about the logistical problems of meeting the needs of very dispersed populations in rural and regional Australia. It was also about government decisions of the past not to increase the government-controlled numbers of general practice training places available (after an increase to 600 nationally in 2004). Thus, while the percentages of rural training pathway acceptances as a proportion of all general practice acceptances had seen a modest increase, the overall numbers of general practitioners had been kept by the previous government at a constant number. Stakeholder data indicated that there was a lack of support for overseas-trained doctors to better orient them to the Australian health system. Stakeholders also expressed concerns about increased demands in the future arising from population trends and increasing expectations on health professionals. They suggested the value of responses such as better incentives for health professionals to work in rural and remote regions and innovative solutions created in partnership with government. The report further advised that workforce policy and planning must engage with factors such as recruitment of medical students from rural areas and the ageing of the health workforce population. It advised that the policy problem of securing better health services for rural and remote areas is not simply about having comparable numbers of health professionals in those regions. It is also about determining what is an adequate workforce configuration for a particular population: the particular mix of health professionals required to meet the needs of a particular community. It concluded that more nuanced responses for particular issues of workforce shortage, such as Aboriginal health workers, were hampered by lack of national data.[77]

Accordingly, this report did not so much offer policy solutions as use existing information to identify what is known and not known about the policy challenges of health workforce shortages in rural and regional Australia. It aimed to clarify the nature of the policy problem facing the Australian government in a context in which there had been considerable 'muddying of the water' by the politics of rural and remote healthcare. The fact that the policy problem had not been clearly understood by the wider Australian community was positioned in this report as not being an accident, but rather the product of political strategy. The report clearly elaborated the importance of previous government decisions in regulating the supply of health practitioners. Yet it also made clear that obtaining an adequate rural and remote workforce required an attention to factors to do with human behaviour in free enterprise systems. As such, it was produced as a 'first step' in the new Rudd government's efforts to design policy solutions to the problem of unequal access to health services in rural and regional Australia.

Chapter 3

Reviewing the evidence

Overview

This chapter identifies critical challenges, tasks, sources, methods, and strategies for doing reviewing in policy-relevant research. It offers exemplars of policy-relevant reviews that extend and highlight this discussion. The aim is to identify possible best practice for such comparative literature analyses, including from the international scholarly literature across the disciplines.

> There is a suspicion between policy-makers and the academic community that maybe the academic community doesn't put all their cards on the table, just the cards that make their case. We all come to our jobs with different points of view and biases and so I think that starting out with an overview of what is known about a topic is actually a very good way for researchers to build their credibility with policy-makers.
>
> (health agency CEO)

Defining the review for health policy

Traditional reviews explore generalizable findings, rather than issues specific to a particular policy context. However, in policy-making contexts, a review is the 'whole process of bringing together a body of evidence which can be drawn from research and other sources, relevant to a particular decision in a policy or management context'[20] (S1:7). In this book, 'the review' as such is conceptualized as a stage that does not involve systematic data collection or community consensus-making exercises. It is about excavation of existing evidence.

The function of the literature review for policy

> . . . you want to tap into the experience that is most similar to yours politically and financially and from a community standpoint. It's important to get the broad perspective; but it's also important to really understand the local perspective as well.
>
> (health agency CEO)

Reviewing in policy-relevant research involves particular practices, both written and social. The emphasis is on sources, in scholarly and other literatures, as well as social sources, that can help the researcher engage with the policy challenges. The broad function of the literature review for policy-relevant research is to help decision-makers see and conceptualize the breadth of issues and broad models that can inform decision-making about the local policy options. However, reviews for policy can be quite different in terms of their specific function which will be defined by the policy problem. Some reviews can be of policy that has remained unchanged for a number of years. Other reviews can involve a policy problem that is likely to emerge in the future if action is not taken.

The review for policy-relevant research involves interpreting and reinterpreting local experience with the policy problem in useful ways that draw on extant sources such as previously published reports, as well as media reports and other already existing information about community views. It also involves examining models in other parts of the country, as well as in different countries, in ways that deliver hard evidence of their compatibility, workability, effectiveness, and value-for-money for the local context. Policy-relevant research is also about in-practice international and national models, weighed for their local workability, including in an economic sense. This genre engages with the challenge of making comparisons of health systems meaningful for 'lesson drawing' for local contexts: a pressing and complex policy learning challenge identified in a growing part of the health policy literature.[78, 79] The review for policy brings together these three kinds of experience and levels of analysis (the local, the national, and the international) in ways that speak to the local policy problems. This involves integrating evidence as diverse as systematic Cochrane reviews and local case studies. To do this the researcher will need to use social skills such as networking and knowledge brokering, as much as analytic research techniques.

> . . . Target the literature review toward all the elements of the policy framework that needs to be enabled by the research, including that issue of cost. Don't limit the literature review to, for example, the biology and the pharmacology of the drug. Extend it to the full pipeline of understanding that's necessary before something gets implemented. 'Extend the literature review all the way to the clinic' might be the best way to describe that.
>
> (health agency CEO)

Challenges in reviewing for health policy

Reviews for policy face challenges that traditional scholarly reviews also face, such as the requirement to make good decisions about what constitutes a good quality versus poor quality study providing evidence of effectiveness. Reviews for health policy also face particular challenges to do with how to, for example,

- synthesize evidence about complex multi-dimensional evidence
- manage process as well as outcome measures
- account for different theories and beliefs about health
- include a wide-ranging set of quantitative and qualitative evidence
- account for unknowns that may have influenced the success of a health intervention or model, such as resources, service delivery quality, and so on.[80]

Key ideas

More broadly, policy-relevant reviews face the major challenge of capturing the contexts of disparate research, and the ways in which those contexts may be similar to, or different from, the specific context of the policy-making challenge for which the review is being conducted.

The scope of the review for health policy

Scholarly health research reviews are often of experimental studies that address questions amenable to such research. They tend not to include studies of other kinds that address broader questions to do with service development that may be of interest to policy-makers.[81] Analyses of how scholarly reviews are conducted suggest that they rarely highlight contextual factors for policy-makers, or offer graded formats that allow easy scanning of the take-home messages for policy-makers, and they frequently present recommendations that may be of dubious value to policy-makers.[81] The focus in these more conventional Cochrane-style reviews on the clinical take-home messages from randomized controlled trials may not best meet the needs of policy-makers.

There are few models of how to use policy-makers in retrospectively adapting the existing body of scholarly review evidence (oriented to global audiences) to meet their local contextual needs.[81] What is known is that scholarly research, as well as many informal information sources, both qualitative and quantitative, must be synthesized in a manner that speaks to policy decision-makers.[20] Not only that; as the last chapter suggested, the review must help decipher the policy problem, including different trade-offs policy-makers might make.[20]

The guidelines for researching for policy-makers published by the Blair government as part of its drive to develop evidence-based policy-making suggest how important it is to develop an 'answerable question' about the policy problem. This should be framed in a manner that will help the researcher deliver a specific answer to this problem, rather than generalized findings:

A systematic review should address a question that has the following four components:

♦ A clear specification of the interventions, factors, or processes in question
♦ A clear specification of the population and/or sub-groups in question
♦ A clear specification of the outcomes that are of interest to the user of the review
♦ A clear specification of the contexts in which the question is set.

An example of an answerable question about a policy intervention might be:

What is the effect of a personal adviser service (intervention) in terms of retaining (outcome 1) and advancing (outcome 2) lone parents (population) in the UK workforce (context)?

An example of an answerable question about the implementation of a policy might be:[82]

What are the barriers (factor/process 1) and facilitating factors (factor/process 2) to getting lone parents (population) to participate (outcome 1) and advance (outcome 2) in the UK workforce (context)?

The aforementioned suggests why interdisciplinary approaches to reviewing, facilitating interactions between the knowledge from different disciplines, are critical to translational research approaches for research-policy transfer.[83] However, researchers may not always be so well equipped to interpret informal or non-scholarly information which may be relevant to a particular policy-making decision.[20] The interdisciplinary and even transdisciplinary nature of policy research requires skills that may not be a part of the training or practical experience of many health researchers.[83] Later sections of this chapter offer tools and approaches for this task.

Context in reviews for health policy

I need to know that the researchers understand the contextual differences between countries, not just the obvious structural differences. I think that's utterly critical . . . it's really hard to know whether such comparative findings are good. I'm still trying to get my country's context, and I'm a citizen . . . . the way policy is made in different countries is really quite different, although on paper they can look relatively similar.

(health agency CEO)

The previous discussion suggests that a critical task of reviewing for policy-making is capturing context-rich evidence that helps policy-makers make effective decisions for their particular populations and systems. What is context in health policy reviews? Dobrow, Goel, and Upshur, a UK and Canada-based health policy research team, have usefully conceptualized two aspects of context. The internal context is about the environment in which a policy decision is made, including the process for decision-making. In contrast, the external context is about the context in which a decision is applied such as disease-specific or political factors which cannot easily be controlled by policy-makers.[34] In practice the two kinds of contexts interact, although the distinction is useful for researchers because it can help them be aware of the different aspects of context about which they will need to collect both formal and informal evidence.

Key ideas

In many health policy contexts it will be critical to not simply explain what works, but rather explain what works, for whom, and in what circumstances. This needs to be done in ways that impart a deeper understanding of relationships between the context in which an intervention has been implemented, the mechanisms that make it work, and the outcomes it produce.[84] This kind of deeper 'realist review' analysis is important to making more nuanced policy decisions about whether a particular intervention will work in a policy context.[84]

Given this, the need to review for context requires the researcher to bring some systemacy to addressing complex contextual issues without also bringing a reductive technical complexity that leaves policy-makers struggling to explain how the conclusions were reached. There is a need to focus on underlying mechanisms that allow the researcher to identify particular permutations of mechanisms that may be successful in particular contexts.[84] The focus in realist reviews for policy is on conceptualizing or theorizing interventions in terms of these underlying mechanisms that influence how and why the intervention works. This involves the researcher for policy bringing together and managing both formal (scholarly published research) and informal (sub-textual, unwritten, off the record, non-scholarly) information and evidence. Later sections of this chapter offer more information about realist review methods. Obviously, the usefulness of the realist review approach is limited by the purpose for which it was designed: evaluating the workability of an intervention.

Sometimes the policy problem is about something else altogether, for example, creating consensus among particular stakeholders on a whole-of-system approach or policy framework.

Using scholarly research

Policy-makers are under pressure to demonstrate that the decisions they make are evidence-based. The available empirical evidence for particular health interventions or service models must be formally assembled with scholarly search methods that stand up to scrutiny by other scholars.[20]

In line with other research, this book emphasizes that epidemiology and clinical research are important to policy-making but may not be so helpful to the theory building that is critical to policy decisions about public health.[85] As suggested previously, the problem of finding local relevance in formal scholarly research is one that policy-makers cite as a barrier to their use of this evidence in policy decision-making.[57] Much formal quantitative evidence used in the United States for public health has been criticized as being too 'medical' in orientation: having a bio-physiological reductionism, a mechanistic quantitative 'black box' approach to data that does not address underlying socio-political causes of health outcomes, preoccupied with identifying individual risk factors or a variable-driven approach to disease, not sufficiently multidisciplinary, and irrelevant to collectivist holistic philosophies of health more in tune with 21st Century needs or health ecologism.[85] This means that formal quantitative studies in the biomedical tradition can be difficult to translate into policy stories about what systemic interventions are needed to achieve systemic outcomes i.e. community-level interventions as opposed to individual patient interventions based on bio-medical notions of causality.[85] At the same time, studies using multi-level statistical modelling of disease offer the promise of more useable basis for exploring the complex multidisciplinary causality of disease useful to 'whole-of-systems' holistic policy-making.[85]

In particular, policy-makers need explicit modelling of decision paths (such as the likelihood of a particular service being used in a particular community) that draw on diverse evidence. They are not helped by attempts to bring a numerical finality (or simplistic 'trust in numbers') to complex information and decision-making situations. The work for policy decision support is often about trying to compare formal information about the performance of other systems. This suffers from problems of comparability within and across systems and the endeavour is beset with difficulties.[86] Extant evidence may also, as for example has been noted of the UK system, be focused on weeding out 'bad apples' rather than yielding up sound information about good performance or identifying best practice.[86]

Key practical strategy

As the tool for deciphering the policy problem suggested in Chapter 2, the limitations in research methods and available data, including scholarly research, are best dealt with by including them as part of the uncertainties accounted for by the researcher.

Many scholarly methods referred to in this book are part of a developing science of decision support modelling and research. Used together they can help achieve the three-dimensional realism and rigour needed for policy support. For example, the science of meta-analysis of the quantitative results of different studies can bring a systemacy to the challenges of review synthesis in a context where narrative methods are perceived as lacking an explicit and easily reproducible method for how the studies were synthesized.[87] But such research will often need to be supplemented by other sources and approaches, such as qualitative research methods.

Using 'grey literature'

> ... in addition to looking at what is going on internationally in your own field, I think it also helps to see what is going on nationally in other fields. . . . Because what is going on nationally in other fields may give you some clues of what will come in the next year or two or three, in your own field.
>
> (health agency CEO)

Research into what kinds of information policy-makers want suggest that they value other sources such as qualitative research, non-randomized quantitative studies, and community reports, all of which do not meet the gold standard for health research.[57] This kind of literature is sometimes called 'grey literature'. A useful study on treating 'grey literature' for policy by Benzies et al. suggests that the grey literature assumes particular importance when the policy option being considered is complex, when there is a lack of consensus about it, particularly in relation to its outcomes, when the context is critical, and when the formal research about the option is limited in amount and quality.[88]

However, grey literature presents particular challenges to do with how it should be treated in best practice reviews, including for health policy.[88] The fact that policy-makers want and need 'grey literature' in their reviews does not of itself mean that such literature can and should be treated in the same way as rigorous randomized clinical trials.

There are two main ways of treating grey literature in research for policy-making. First, grey literature can be used to supplement and triangulate information from the empirical scholarly literature that meets the gold standard for evidence. For example, the use of case studies in reviews presents particular challenges because they are not generalizable in the statistical sense but rather have an internal validity that relates to the coherence of the theoretical reasoning.[89, 90] Yet case studies grey literature can be valuable when used to supplement randomized controlled trials in ways that help in the theory building so important to policy arguments.

Another example is testimony from public enquiry websites—independent reviews of public policy—common in the United Kingdom, Canada, and Australia, but not so much in the United States. There are some useful papers on how to treat these sorts of sources.[91] They can offer information that helps triangulate what the scholarly (and other grey literature) literature is saying, for example in relation to unusual cases such as hospital error.

A second way of treating grey literature is by way of using it to trace the experience of a community and its policy-makers with a particular policy problem. This kind of document analysis is a critical task in reviewing for health policy. Consultancy reports, briefings, and other material produced by local and other organizations are often important to understanding the history surrounding a policy problem. Media and other accounts of the reception of these community-based reports can also be valuable to understanding what actually happened to the proposals in such reports, why. Searching community and media accounts to examine the history of a policy challenge can be challenging because the same policy arguments may be couched in quite different language (and different language can be used to describe the same policy problem). Chapter 4 on designing research methods highlights the value of discourse analysis as a qualitative approach to engaging with the complexities of language when analysing the policy problem. Document analysis also features in the Blair government's resources for delivering better evidence to policy-makers: readers should consult *The Magenta Book* for an introduction to the concept.[82]

Key practical strategy

In practice, the two approaches to treating grey literature are not mutually exclusive. For example, document analysis of grey literature can be used to not only triangulate the evidence in the gold standard scholarly literature but also to trace the experience of a local community with a particular policy problem.

Information from policy networks

Information from informal networks such as contacts in health agencies or clinician networks can be critical to triangulating possibly out-of-date information from reports of system outcomes based on quantitative data. Such informal information may not be so valuable for presentation in formal reports because it may be biased and hard to aggregate.[86] It may also have been given to the researcher 'off the record'. The challenge is for the researcher to utilize networks for getting this informal information, so that it can help illuminate power relationships and struggles that made a particular intervention in a particular context sink or swim.[84]

Key practical strategy

The real value of information from policy networks lies in its use helping the researcher reflect on how to avoid using apparently correct 'hard' data incorrectly. Informal information from policy networks can be helpful to identifying areas where apparently correct 'hard data' must be supplemented with further formal research investigations that are reportable.

Accordingly, a key challenge in policy-relevant research is often designing an approach to gathering this 'soft intelligence'. In health systems, like other systems, there will be cultural barriers to the 'free-flow of soft intelligence' to do with the incentives that operate to encourage silence about, for example, under-performance[86] (p.17).

How can policy networks be identified and used? In *Using Evidence: How Research can Inform Public Services* Nutley, Walter, and Davies identify four key types of networks suggested by the research literature:

- ◆ 'policy communities' which include both academics and analysts within and beyond government who have specialist experience and knowledge of a particular policy area and are well-integrated into a particular policy-making process
- ◆ 'advocacy coalitions' which comprise a broad range of stakeholders in the private, public, and not-for-profit sectors which are formed on the basis of shared beliefs
- ◆ 'epistemic communities' comprised of experts with technical and scientific knowledge in a particular area relevant to health policy-making
- ◆ 'issue networks' which are fluid and ad hoc networks comprised of people who have formed a coalition on the basis of a particular issue.[36]

Researchers for policy may wish to reflect on the different kinds of networks that may be relevant to their contexts. Available written documents on the policy issues can include contacts that offer a useful point of departure for assembling a map of policy networks, prior to getting input from key people.

Search strategies

Practical guides and tools for reviewing for policy-makers

Researchers for policy might want to search for up-to-date models, guides, and protocols for qualitative searches in particular.[20, 87, 92] The quality guides available for conducting reviews for policy-makers emphasize the importance not only of systematic searches of scholarly databases, and scholarly conference proceedings, but also searches of the internet, use of networks (not just with other researchers) and so on.[20] A useful summary of strategies for high quality reviews for public health is given by Waters et al.[80] It points out that the relatively tightly organized and accessible nature of bio-medical literature contrasts with the more sprawling and multidisciplinary nature of public health studies involving a wider range of bibliographical tools and terminology. Reviewers for public health policy may thus need to obtain a substantial proportion of their references from talking with contacts.[80]

Reviewers for public health policy can consult resource centres offering guidance. Through its Public Health Research Group, the Cochrane Collaboration offers a model for how to do reviews for public health policy which focuses more on the needs of public health policy-makers (http://www.vichealth.vic.gov.au). This model is characterized by an emphasis on policy questions and concerns: a process for ensuring input for end users of the review at different stages of development; a broader focus on the effects of healthcare interventions; and use, where necessary, of narrative synthesis of study results, as well as meta-analysis.[80] There is also a Cochrane Qualitative Methods Network which offers models of how to treat qualitative research in ways that supplement Cochrane reviews of randomized controlled trials (http://www.joannabriggs.edu.au). The NHS Centre for Reviews and Dissemination also offers the results of systematic reviews focussing on the outcomes of health and social care interventions, including economic evaluations of health interventions, and enquiries into information dissemination (http://www.york.ac.uk). The Evidence for Policy and Practice Information and Co-ordinating Centre (EPPI-Centre) in London suggests the same emphasis on systematic reviews for policy making, but in the social sciences, though it does also treat health promotion (http://eppi.ioe.ac.uk). The ESRC UK Centre for Evidence-based Policy and Practice also provides resources for researchers and policy-makers, including plain language summaries and studies of best practice in doing research for policy-makers (http://www.esrcsocietytoday.ac.uk/ESRCInfoCentre). The website of the Centre for Reviews and Dissemination at the University of York offers quite detailed guidelines about how to construct protocols for reviews. However, these will need to be adapted for a particular local policy-making context (http://www.york.ac.uk). The Campbell Collaboration is an international organization that acts as a conduit of research evidence for policy-makers. It places a strong emphasis on reviews of largely experimental/quasi-experimental trials conducted in the social policy-making areas outside health. However, some relevant fields are also included such as the education of healthcare professionals, and of course, many areas of social research such as crime prevention have multidisciplinary value for health services policy-making (http://www.campbellcollaboration.org/).

In the United States there are a host of health policy research centres: the Resource Center for Health Policy at the University of Washington (http://depts.washington.edu); the UCLA Center for Health Policy Research (http://www.healthpolicy.ucla.edu); the Center for Health Policy at Duke University (http://www.hpolicy.duke.edu). These can act as useful conduits of American health policy research practices. Researchers should also consult the resources included on the web pages of such organizations as The Coalition for Evidence-Based Policy which is a non-profit, non-partisan organization sponsored by the Council for Excellence in Government which aims to develop evidence-based policy-making through advocacy, though in fields beyond health (http://www.excelgov.org).

Different government departments have developed standards for the production of research. For example, in the United Kingdom, the Department of Health has developed a national health research strategy 'Best Research for Health' (http://www.dh.gov.uk). There is much value in examining what is shaping government policy makers' views of good evidence-based decision-making. The characteristics of modern evidence-based decision-making in the public service have been described particularly within the United Kingdom, for example, in the UK Government's publication *Professional Policy Making for the 21st Century*.[44] Websites for policy-makers aimed at encouraging evidence-based decision-making can also be very helpful to researchers for policy, such as the Policy Hub, a UK government website (http://www.nationalschool.gov.uk/policyhub).

In the United States, Congress requires that all federal agencies must meet performance measures that assess the success of interventions. These involve three types of measures related to programme success:

1 Output measures relating to the volume of work achieved such as the number of clients etc.

2 Outcome measures to do with the consequences of a programme or intervention such as reduction in reported instances of particular health conditions.

3 Efficiency measures to do with the effect of the project on an agency's efficiency in relation to its resource use, for example, the cost of particular health services.

The United States Office of Management and Budget (OMB) has developed guidelines for assessing the performance of federal programmes government-wide. These include The Programme Assessment Rating Tool (PART) which has been developed by OMB for the purposes of assessing and improving programme performance (http://www.whitehouse.gov). Associated guidance documents reinforce the view that randomized controlled trials remain the gold standard for evaluations, especially in high stakes health areas. However, a range of other quasi-experimental and non-experimental approaches may often also need to be used.[93]

Such standards informing performance measures and models of 'performance metrics' for different interventions around the world offer a point of departure for reflecting on how to gather and synthesize information about 'what works'.

Developing judgments about the quality of evidence for policy

Many guidelines operating in health research have the limitations for policy-making identified by Pawson i.e. imposing a single hierarchy of quality does not allow the widest possible range of formal and informal information to be included to build up the mosaic picture that the policy problem will require.[84] In fact, some policy-makers may not value or want approaches that are informed by such scholarly rankings of the 'rigour' of research because the 'higher' levels of evidence do not provide the information decision-makers need.[57] As Pawson rightly argues, the worth of studies for complex policy-making contexts does not lie in establishing their *a priori* value, but rather in the synthesis and weighing up of their relevance for consideration of a particular policy problem.[84] Reliance solely on hierarchical protocols that privilege a notion of quality implicit in randomized controlled trials will often not allow the researcher to engage with the evidence needs of policy-makers.

However, it may be critical when a biomedical matter requires clarification to be informed by traditional Cochrane-style notions of quality that sharply distinguish randomized controlled trials from grey literature or informal information such as advice in textbooks.[87] It is often the case that some aspects of the policy problem may involve sequestering off randomized controlled trials to offer an empirical clinical answer.

How should qualitative papers be judged for health policy research? A useful paper by Popay, Rogers, and Williams on the rationale and standards for systematic treatment of qualitative research in health services research offers one kind of answer. It suggests that good qualitative research is defined by three inter-related criteria by which it can be judged across its different areas, from theoretical base to sampling strategy to scope of data collection to data analysis, to its output. The three areas are:

1 The interpretation of subjective meanings: good qualitative research illuminates the meanings that people give to their experiences.

2 The description of wider social context: good qualitative research captures rich contextual information.

3 An attention to lay people's knowledge.[92]

For example, while the presence of randomized treatment control groups and statistical power is critical to notions of quality informing classical experimental designs, sampling for qualitative studies should be assessed on the extent to which it delivers on the three aforementioned criteria.[92]

The UK Government's Cabinet Office has also developed a framework for assessing qualitative research that is particularly suitable for reviewing for policy-making contexts. It provides appraisal questions and quality indicators based on four in-principle criteria for assessing qualitative research: whether the research contributes to the field of knowledge, has a defensible design fit for its purpose, is rigorously (systematically and transparently) conducted, and makes credible claims.[94]

Key practical strategy

Notions of quality informing policy research will ideally be informed by a 'fitness for purpose' test, in which the complex set of considerations for policy may require different kinds of evidence and different standards of quality for treating that evidence. In making selections of scholarly evidence, scholarly notions of quality certainly can help make distinctions based on inferences about quality. The different schema that exist for assessing the quality of scholarly evidence, from quantitative randomized controlled trials to qualitative case studies,[20, 87] should be presented in the policy-relevant report in ways that convey those differences. Yet the lack of criteria for quality that can be applied to *both* quantitative and qualitative scholarly research means that the researcher will need to adapt these protocols in ways that make sense for the policy problem being examined.

Search techniques

Searches for formal literature will probably involve a number of databases, one in conjunction with another, using purposive and snowballing techniques as well as other techniques to test particular interpretations of the wider body of literature.[84] Yet, as has been noted, even when the policy-relevant researcher is targeting scholarly journals, it will be important to talk with contacts in the field—not just other researchers, but also policy-makers and stakeholders—to ensure that the review includes the kinds of formal evidence and information that has currency in policy contexts. Networking will also be critical to identifying and understanding population health databases, and any associated studies using these databases. The details of precisely how particular databases held by, for example, the Australian Bureau of Statistics, are constructed, can often only be obtained through direct contact with those researchers involved in constructing the survey items and the internal logic of the databases.

Often the search techniques used will be pragmatic: searches of vaster expanses of non-scholarly material until saturation point or the researcher is finding nothing new.[20] Grey literature should be sorted and sifted through in ways that allow it to be used to develop the external validity (the usefulness for policy-makers and the community) of the review for policy-making. Questions that can be asked to select sources are: 'How relevant is this study to the local contextual policy problem being examined?' and 'What can policy-makers say with what level of confidence using this study?'

Key practical strategy

Where the bibliographic information, both formal and informal, is likely to be vast, it may be helpful to begin with a 'scoping review' to establish the extent and nature of references needed. A scoping review is a quick scan and description of sources that allows the researcher to develop a sense of how much and what kinds of research and information, formal and informal, will need to be excavated. This can be very helpful in policy-making contexts, which typically presents researchers with tight timelines. Any decisions about setting search parameters can be made once this has been done.[95]

Chapter 2 referred to the value of using a table categorizing 'certainties' and 'uncertainties' about the policy problem. Once developed in working draft form, this tool can also be used to aid search techniques for, and conceptual development of, the review. That is, the information supplied by the review can be used to modify the table, and the table can be used to develop directions for reviewing.

Synthesising the information for review

Scholarly literature suggests a broad range of tools for synthesising different kinds of evidence in reviews for health policy-making. Researchers who know about these possibilities are well-positioned to develop an approach that works for their context. For example, there are narrative approaches, approaches that variously translate all the evidence into either qualitative or quantitative form, Bayesian meta-analysis and decision analysis that converts qualitative evidence into quantitative syntheses, and approaches that translate quantitative study findings into quantitative syntheses (meta-analysis).[20]

In weighing the different methods, the researcher will want to consider the expectations of policy-makers. For example, sometimes policy-makers contract researchers because they want expert advice on a particular topic. Other times they want the researcher to provide generic research skills that will deliver a description of the evidence. Such expectations of policy-makers may shape the choice and delivery of the method of synthesis of the review, such as the way a narrative approach is employed or the use of statistical methods.

Each method has it strengths and weaknesses for a particular policy-making context. It is not the purpose of this book to identify and describe the different review approaches that can be employed; they are as diverse as research itself. The discussion that follows highlights some possible approaches to synthesizing information for the policy-relevant review.

Qualitative methods for reviewing

Narrative qualitative methods for reviewing have the advantage that they do not require technical transformation of the evidence—information collected by the review to be transformed into metrics.[20] However, delivering such an approach competently does require high level analytical and writing skills of policy story-telling, and a capacity to speak to the underlying policy issues. Some narrative approaches have been identified in a helpful paper by Mays, Pope, and Popay on reviewing techniques for researchers for policy-makers.[20]

Key ideas

Narrative approaches can all suffer from a perceived lack of objectivity because the researcher often has arranged the material under different themes or concepts to tell the policy story and thus may not be able to offer a technical-numerical explanation of the method used to arrive at the conclusions.[20] This concern is not just that of empirically minded scholars engaged in territory wars. It is also raised in the applied public sector literature such as the work on best practice in delivering evidence to policy-makers produced by the Blair government.[82] If a narrative approach is chosen, policy-makers will expect that the researcher's opinions of the evidence will be clearly distinguished from the facts as they are known.

Clearly, different kinds of sources may require different kinds of narrative frameworks for reading them. For example, discourse analysis is a form of structured, qualitative, language-centred analysis that can be useful to considering documents offering testimonies in public enquiries.[91] However, great care has to be exercised when interpreting such testimonies as they are typically excerpts from larger transcriptions: all the relevant conditions under which they were collected and the nature of other information supplied in the testimony from individuals is rarely known.[91] More details are given in the next chapter under the section on qualitative methods—strictly speaking discourse analysis is more a research method than a technique for reviewing as such. The point being made here is that no narrative method, no matter how sophisticated, can overcome a lack of basic information about those texts.

The section on context in reviewing suggested that an important policy-relevant method for reviewing that relies on narrative forms is the 'realist review' associated with Pawson and colleagues.[84] This analyses the context in which an intervention has been applied more deeply than traditional reviewing methods, aiming to deliver better explanation of how complex programmes work in particular situations.[84] It also involves utilizing social networks to obtain 'off the record' information about the contextual conditions operating in other systems with respect to particular interventions. Accordingly, the realist researcher will use a wide range of primary sources.[84]

There are two basic activities in a realist review approach, as outlined by Pawson and colleagues in their paper 'Realist review—a new method of systematic review designed for complex policy interventions'.[84] The first activity is generating a comprehensive theory of the social and other conditions under which interventions work, using multiple formal and informal sources to create a mosaic picture of causality. The second is generating conclusions in a format that describes what interventions work under what conditions: exploring the answers to 'why', 'when', and 'how' questions.[84, 96] The complexity of the questions addressed by a realist review mean that the reviewing process will be much more iterative. This is not simply in terms of the assembling of written information but also in the involvement of policy-makers and stake-holders to help clarify the focus of the research. At the very least, the focus of the realist review method on mapping underlying mechanisms that make interventions work in particular contexts can be used in policy-relevant reviews to ensure that they do not focus on irrelevant detail. Wading through vast amounts of literature on the effectiveness of this or that intervention requires a sort logic. Realist narrative can give the researcher this sort logic: as Pawson says, it is more a review logic or 'a logic of discovery' than a review technique.[84]

Another thematic approach to reviewing, mentioned earlier, is the 'scoping study' which departs from the typical Cochrane review in the sense that it addresses broader topics and is more inclusive of different kinds of study designs.[95] It also includes working with stakeholders and networks to obtain access to a wide range of informal information. It may have particular value as an approach to not simply creating a preliminary map of the literature, but also summarizing the literature for the purpose of disseminating it to policy-makers. This method can involve charting and sorting material according to key themes and issues, using a database program.[95] The information charted for policy-relevant research can be general information about the study as well as specific information such as methodology, outcomes measures and results[95], and so on, which can be helpful to deciphering and resolving the policy problem. The results are not synthesized as such as in a traditional systematic review where 'quality' studies are emphasized. Rather, the scoping review aims to map the extent, nature, and distribution of studies using tables and charts: the geographical and care groups they relate to, range of interventions, research methods, measures of effectiveness, and so on.[95] Many variations of this kind of scoping study are possible, including mapping research by competing approaches to a particular policy challenge. Such maps can include information helpful to assessing the 'weight of evidence' that can be given to each study, even though quality appraisal is not the primary purpose of the scoping method.[95]

Another approach to synthesizing non-experimental studies should be mentioned here, not least because it has been highlighted in UK government resources for delivering research to policy-makers; 'meta-ethnography'.[82] Meta-ethnography is an interpretative, narrative method that offers strategies for synthesizing qualitative studies. It takes a social and cultural explanatory focus through the use of metaphors. An example of its application in health may be to the challenge of reviewing studies of organizational culture in the clinical error literature. Meta-ethnography shares the perceived shortcomings of other narrative methods that do not offer quantification of their findings. However, its supporters might argue that meta-ethnography is about identifying patterns of consistency and inconsistency rather than numerical summaries.[82] Readers might like to consult the foundation text for this method, *Meta-Ethnography: Synthesizing Qualitative Studies* by Noblit and Hare.[97]

The discussion of scoping reviews suggested that researchers for policy-makers can tabulate all data thematically in both quantitative and qualitative forms. Qualitative data can be tabulated for reviewing purposes when, for example, considering multiple case studies of related but different phenomena. However, qualitative data from reviews can also be converted into quantitative form. For example, this can happen when using a method known as 'content analysis' which at its simplest level involves counting frequencies of particular things in texts using explicit rules for coding.[20] However, such tabulation and frequency counts need to be used cautiously, as they can lose contextual richness while delivering little by way of rigorous summary methods.

Quantitative methods for reviewing

Bayesian meta-analysis and quantitative decision analysis can be used to convert all data into quantitative form which can then be analysed and modelled.[20] Simulations of effectiveness, including cost effectiveness, can then be obtained delivering models of decision-making paths using weights and probabilities.[20] More discussion of such methods is given in the next chapter. Some key issues in reviewing using quantitative methods are highlighted here.

The most accepted method for reviewing using quantitative methods is meta-analysis. Meta-analysis for reviewing involves statistical treatment of quantitative results to summarize the results from different studies, both randomized controlled trials and non-randomized studies.[87] The details of this method has been exhaustively documented elsewhere: readers might like to consult *Systematic Reviews in Health Care.* [98] Meta-analysis has brought systemacy to reviewing and has been effective in bringing evidence to bear on a number of prevailing health myths.[99] Its limitations for policy-making are that it does not engage with the broad range of qualitative evidence that might count, the contexts of the studies so analysed or that of the policy-makers for whom the meta-analysis is being done.

Pawson has criticized meta-analysis for the way it is based on bio-medical research models, eliminating the critical explanatory content and causal complexity of different interventions to arrive at a seeming rigour of *arithmetic* summary via simplification, standardization and aggregation (he argues that narrative methods also reduce complexity to simplifications of what is generally true).[96, 100] However, meta-analysis may have value for considering the weight of evidence on bio-medical matters that are part of the health policy problem.

Making choices about methods for synthesizing information

Key ideas

Researchers can select a combination of different approaches to synthesizing literature to tailor-make the review to meet the specific needs of a policy-maker. Critical considerations are ensuring that the reviewing methods used allow the policy story to be told in the review simply and clearly for non-technical audiences and in time to meet the policy-making deadlines.

Many reviews for policy need to be completed in 2 or 3 months, which is much shorter than the normal 6 months allowed for major systematic scholarly reviews. This is why other approaches to reviewing have been developed, such as the Health Technology Assessments (HTAs). Health Technology Assessments answer some basic questions about health interventions such as clinical outcomes, impact on quality and length of life, costs and savings, in a descriptive manner oriented to the needs of the United Kingdom's NHS policy-making.[97]

The choice and use of methods for synthesizing the review must also meet another critical aim: triangulation of the different kinds of evidence, especially in relation to potentially high stakes decision-making. 'Triangulation' is described more fully in the next chapter. It is also important in reviewing to ensure that different kinds of evidence are used to add to the robustness and completeness of the evidence for policy.

Observational data and qualitative case study data can also be used to complement and supplement randomized controlled trials in ways that build conceptual frameworks for the policy story.[90] This movement from the concrete to the abstract, from biomedical and structural explanations to explanations of social agency, not just at the review stage, but at all stages of the research as it unfolds, is part of the art of policy story-telling described in Chapter 7.[90]

Recommended reading

Pawson R, Tilley N. *Realistic Evaluation*. London, Sage Publications, 2000.

Case studies in reviewing for health policy

Case study: reviewing the evidence for communicable disease policy and programme development in Singapore

Singapore has made substantial efforts in the area of communicable disease 'surveillance' or the ongoing collection and analysis of population data aimed at identifying the nature, extent, and trends in communicable diseases. This effort aims to provide a basis for the development of policy and interventions, including as part of a prevention approach, to communicable diseases.

The report Communicable Disease Surveillance in Singapore 2007[101] can be considered part of this effort. Produced on an annual basis, it offers a compilation of epidemiological data obtained through the Ministry of Health's partnerships with medical professionals. As such it is most useful at the level of formulating population health policy.

The report analyses population data for air/droplet-borne disease, vector-borne/zoonotic diseases, food/water-borne disease, environment-related diseases, HIV/AIDS, sexually transmitted diseases, tuberculosis, and leprosy based on notifications by medical professionals.

Different kinds of data from different agencies and sources, involving different styles of data analyses were used. The report offers visual representations of the data using readily accessible formats: tables, bar and line charts, as well as maps of Singapore offering spatial representations of population health data.

The report also includes special features and case studies of specific instances of communicable disease control and management useful to reflecting on policy. For example, it includes an analysis of an outbreak of salmonellosis. This synthesizes information about departmental management of an outbreak of this condition, including the results of health inspections, as well as clinical information, epidemiological and microbiological analyses, and selected research literature. The report then offers three major policy implications of the case study: measures for ensuring food handlers are practicing appropriate hygiene; that certain foods (cream cakes) could be considered high risk items that require more stringent microbiological testing; better inventory systems for tracing ingredients and products useful to product recall.

The primary value of the report is thus as a snapshot or overview of population health status in relation to communicable diseases in Singapore, identifying 'big picture' population health issues. It compresses much diverse information to offer an accessible tool for annual review by Singaporean health policy-makers. The implications of the information it presents are both retrospective (how did we manage what happened?) as well as prospective (what trends suggest where our efforts would be best spent?).

Case study: Australia: The healthiest country by 2020 a discussion paper

In September 2008 the federal government of Australia released a discussion paper on preventative health that focussed on obesity, tobacco, and alcohol consumption—Australia: The Healthiest Country by 2020 A Discussion Paper.[102] The discussion paper was developed by a taskforce set up in April 2008 by the Australian government. It aimed to stimulate public discussion prior to the development of a comprehensive preventative health strategy for Australia in 2009.

The body of the discussion paper offered a synthesis of scholarly and applied literature on Australia's health outcomes and the case for prevention, particularly in relation to obesity, tobacco, and alcohol-related challenges. It included:

* population health data from Australia, including health-related behaviours, and related epidemiology studies, which in turn included comparative international surveys from such agencies as the Organization for Economic Cooperation and Development (OECD)

* the results of scholarly and applied literature on health prevention as it relates to obesity, tobacco, and alcohol consumption; this included the results of initiatives in other countries, English and non-English-speaking

* the results of predictive analyses for health outcomes, national and comparative international trends

* legislative, regulatory, and policy developments and models in the field of health prevention, in public and private sectors, as well as comparative international analyses of such developments and models, gleaned from a range of sources including media reports

* quotable information from reputable sources such as the World Health Organization

◆ retrospective and prospective information about health costs and benefits—the 'knock on' costs of health-harming behaviours and the benefits of interventions targeting them—including from applied research studies conducted by government departments as well as international comparative studies.

The information in the main report was arranged around layperson's questions such as 'Why the focus on obesity, tobacco, and alcohol?' As such, the purpose of the discussion paper was to help develop informed debate about the health prevention challenges facing Australia.

The report did more than argue that obesity, tobacco, and alcohol consumption presented major present and future challenges to Australians' health. It also argued that these three factors had a major role to play in producing health inequities between rich and poor, indigenous and non-indigenous, rural and urban Australians. It presented the evidence that prevention was the key to making a difference to the health of Australians, especially disadvantaged communities. More than that, it articulated the conceptual framework for, and argued for the value of, a particular kind of approach to health prevention: a 'whole-of-community' approach targeting population-level behaviour changes that involves effective regulation and legislation as well as effective and sustained public education. It also identified barriers to prevention such as economic market interests and forces.

The main report also identified the major actions, particularly at the national level, needed to address obesity, tobacco, and alcohol consumption, such as protecting children from inappropriate marketing of unhealthy comestibles. It included suggestions about relevant performance indicators and related processes for performance monitoring and evaluation. Questions were embedded in the report to help prompt community feedback, and guidelines for the content of community submissions were included.[102]

Three technical reports were appended to the main report: one each for obesity, tobacco, and alcohol consumption.[103–105] These provided the detail of directions for action and supporting research that was summarized in the main report. References to sources were used to synthesize the key conclusions about 'what works', as well as identify the unknowns of obesity, tobacco, and alcohol consumption, and draw out related policy implications. In particular these technical reports helped substantiate the main policy argument that obesity, tobacco, and alcohol consumption perpetuate social disadvantage that prevention can help overcome.

This Australian example of reviewing for health policy demonstrates some key characteristics of the genre. For example, such reviews can be used to explore a particular set of policy problems as the first step in community consensus-building for policy options. They typically draw on very diverse multidisciplinary information, qualitative and quantitative, presented in accessible formats for more general readers. This information may include the up-to-date policy decisions of agencies that are not so well-documented in the scholarly literature. Technical information may be appended; however, scholarly rigour and a valuing of authoritative sources underpins the apparent populist nature of such reports.

Chapter 4

Designing research methods for health policy

Overview

This chapter highlights some key approaches in designing research methods for health policy: the critical issues of validity and credibility, as well as key features of innovative approaches to health policy decision support.

Challenges in designing research methods for health policy

> . . . if I'm talking about policies which have to do with clinical standards of the provision of care, then I think being very clear and being very thorough about the scientific evidence for a particular issue is absolutely critical . . . But if I had to look at the non-clinical healthcare policy, for example, administration or maybe manpower planning, which has less of a patient-in-the-face component, then I think something that's more implementable, more pragmatic in its approach, would be something that I would prefer to see.
>
> (health agency CEO)

Research methods for health policy-makers present specific challenges. There is no one method that 'works', because each method has different strengths and weaknesses for delivering policy-relevant research. Different research techniques from different disciplines can help add value to ways of doing policy-relevant research. Considered collectively, the work of scholars from these different disciplines offers strategies for overcoming the weaknesses of traditional quantitative and qualitative methods for health policy contexts and bringing a much-needed methodological inventiveness to policy-relevant research.

As the last chapter suggested, classical statistical methods have a critical role to play in obtaining information for macro-social policy in large-N, variable-driven analyses, but they have some important limitations for 21st century health policy agendas. They have value in clinical experimental studies in the traditional bio-medical model but have their limits for the holistic challenges of contemporary healthcare policy and practice: in countering the regional health effects of climate change, in health prevention efforts aimed at tackling the socio-economic determinants of health, in healthy ageing and chronic disease, in adolescent risk-taking linking health, education and welfare, in ecologically-influenced childhood conditions such as asthma, in providing equal access to affordable healthcare services, in health services quality assurance and clinical error, as well as many other areas. The health policy challenges of today require research paradigms that integrate bio-psycho-social factors. More than that, many health policy challenges require research that engages with client-service-community interactions, including in small-N contexts of political significance for policy-makers, such as those found in rural and remote communities. Quantitative techniques may have good internal validity, but they often lack external validity for complex service settings, limiting their value for policy-relevant research. On the other hand, qualitative approaches associated with ethnography, social reproduction, hermeneutics, and critical discourse theory, may lead to a focus on capturing the ecological complexity of healthcare settings at the expense of reliability and generalizability. This produces results of limited value for high stakes policy decision-making. In a culture of 'trust in numbers' and political spin, policy-relevant research must be both highly numerate and strategically literate.

Key ideas

The art of designing research methods for health policy lies in adapting and combining different qualitative and quantitative techniques to meet the evidence needs of policy-making where particular notions of causality, bias, and rigour apply. Designing research for policy is about seeing how different techniques can complement and supplement one another, rather than adhering to narrow ideas about quantitative or qualitative research.

There are many possibilities in policy-relevant research for combinatorial research designs, from linking elements of cost effectiveness research and decision analysis with clinical trials to linking mathematical modelling in operational research with qualitative methods for community participation. What matters in policy-relevant research is the fitness for purpose of the method for what is often an exercise in systemic interventions to achieve systemic outcomes with social collectivist, rather than individual, dimensions.[85]

Policy-relevant research is also likely to face challenges of integrating methods for evaluating the cost-effectiveness of different emerging health policy options in ways that will be persuasive to the wider community. These are methods for evaluating not only different kinds of action, but also the costs of inaction, in a 'money talks' policy world needing simple predictive economic modelling allowing comparison of the 'best buys'.

Combining different methods allows the results of one method to be used to triangulate findings from another method. Triangulation is a critical challenge of designing research for policy-makers, including where randomization is impossible.[106] It involves using the findings of one method, kind of data, investigator, or theory to cross-check the findings of another method, kind of data, investigator, or theory.[82] The higher the policy decision-making stakes, the greater the need for triangulation.

In using combinatorial research designs, researchers for health policy aim to meet strongly contextual evidence needs, whether they relate to macro policy-making (where large-N population data is critical such as healthcare rebate policies), meso policy-making (where aggregated data must have regional service design value), or micro policy-making (where small-N data is critical, as in local community health prevention). Macro, meso, and micro policy-making all share challenges to do with getting diversity-oriented evidence that integrates information from both large-N and small-N datasets.

In policy-relevant research, it is important to first determine what the nature of the policy problem is before deciding what method to use: does it require 'street level observations' that may require an operational research approach, or does it require prospective cost effectiveness modelling of different services, or does it require rigorous experimental data about drug efficacy? Therefore, before reaching a decision about what method to use, researchers may first want to consider not simply the research questions, but the specific hypotheses that need to be tested.

These kinds of challenges are the focus of this chapter.

Intelligent design for policy

. . . health systems certainly are very difficult to define through hypothesis-driven research. The systems seem to change too quickly. And I wonder sometimes whether the classic scientific methods of defining hypothesis holding conditions stable and changing one variable, whether the training that many science folks engaged in health policies . . . That background, that training is sometimes not useful in terms of understanding the descriptive methodologies, and the quality improvement methodologies that tend to inform policy. You know people with scientific background tend to look for that hypothesis during research, and when it's not there they say the material's not useful. And that's a real problem.

So if you look at quality improvement literature, for example, with its heavy emphasis on what I tend to call the 'small tests of change' as a way of understanding system transformation and improvement in systems, the folks who have a hypothesis-driven-controlled-study-methodology background cannot appreciate the more qualitative approach to quality improvement techniques.

(health agency CEO)

A key feature of quality research for health policy lies in its 'intelligent design' for local contextual needs. It is not enough to translate the policy challenges into policy problems and then 'research questions'. Specific hypotheses often need to be tested. However, hypothesis testing in policy-relevant research has a particular nature. It can be quite different from what is narrowly understood as a scientific hypothesis in classical experimental studies. It often involves testing specific assumptions implicit in understanding the policy problem, whether they derive from policy-makers or the wider community, or the media. Such assumptions can be tested in ways that allow the researcher to question them effectively in the interests of community debate and health reform. The quantitative and qualitative research designs developed should be capable of performing such tests, and of triangulating the evidence for critical hypotheses, as well as identifying unknown policy problems. There will also be specific issues of political face-value validity and credibility of evidence that matter to policy-makers, which will need to be included in the research design. This will shape how the hypotheses for policy should be tested.

Validity and credibility in policy-relevant research

There are two aspects of validity that matter in policy-relevant research: internal validity and external validity. Internal validity relates to the research rigour: the extent to which the design reflects efforts to remove human distortions and bias through such efforts as randomized treatment control groups, and rigorous statistical techniques.[107] Internal validity is about the extent to which the study findings are, technically speaking, generalizable to a particular population. This relates to the sampling techniques used.

Key practical strategy

An introductory discussion of sampling for policy-making research is given in *The Magenta Book* produced by the Cabinet Office of the Blair government.[82] It suggests that any policy-relevant questions to do with the nature and precision of estimates, differences between subgroups, changes over time, and so on will need to be worked out in advance in consultation with policy-makers.[82]

External validity relates to the extent to which the research findings are meaningful to a community of users of those findings, such as policy-makers and practitioners. This notion of validity involves another idea of generalizability of findings that is about what is meaningful not for researchers, but for policy-makers and practitioners.[107] For example, unless particular professional groups are included the findings may have no political credibility and therefore no robust external validity (although a random sampling method may suggest that technically speaking the findings are representative). These kinds of political credibility issues are explored further in Chapter 6 on consensus-building for health policy.

The exhortation in the policy literature to involve community members and policy-makers in the design of the research is partly about trying to achieve this external validity. The fact that policy-makers must make high stakes decisions that are meaningful to their contexts means researchers for policy cannot neglect either notion of validity. In practice though, trade-offs must be made between internal and external validity. This will shape decisions about research design which is ultimately about fitness for purpose.

Using experimental research designs: accommodating complex causality

The first thing that researchers need to do is very carefully describe the patient population in the study: who are you actually describing? Secondly, research needs to define whether or not there is a clinically significant improvement—the evaluation of the intervention . . . in other words, has it truly made a difference: is that difference just a statistical reality or is it something that's actually clinically significant? The third thing is the description of cost effectiveness: that's always useful in terms of understanding what the outcome is and whether or not it is worthy of implementation . . . It's not good enough to demonstrate that intervention A causes a better outcome than intervention B; it's also crucially important to look at all the other aspects of quality of care: how does this impact on the delivery of care, how does it impact on the patient's satisfaction related to care, how does it impact crucially on the cost of care? These are issues that the researcher should be thinking about if they're interested in translating their research, in basic research making an impact. They have to think through 'how would it be implemented?'

(health agency CEO)

As the introduction in particular suggested, the scholarly literature includes a growing chorus of voices that point to the chasm between the body of evidence arising from clinical trials and the needs of policy and practice. Part of the reason for this chasm may be the design of experimental trials and the nature of the evidence they produce. For example, the criteria used by most medical and healthcare journals to guide authors are based on checklists of internal validity that place little emphasis on external validity.[108] The role of randomized controlled trials in much of health research has privileged particular notions of research quality to do with the internal validity of experimental research designs and associated quantitative approaches. Explanations of phenomena under study (causality) in health research have often been about identifying variables of interest in ways that meet these 'internal' or 'within-experimental-research-design' criteria for quality.[109] As Steven Lewis has wittily surmised, the growing literature on the limitations of randomized controlled trials for holistic 'real world' decision-making suggests the value of being aware of 'the unbearable lightness of being statistically correct' [110] (p. 166).

In contrast, policy-makers (and practitioners) often require holistic evidence that is useable in their specific local context i.e. has 'external validity' for them.[109] In fact, causality as it is defined in classical experimental studies may not be so important in policy decision-making which is more concerned with effectiveness in specific 'real world' contexts.[106] Thus, evidence-based policy-making requires developing existing research methods, techniques, and ideas about causality, validity, and so on, to achieve external validity for policy-making contexts. As this book has emphasized, randomized clinical trials and the traditional statistical methods associated with them can have poor utility for policy-makers because they often do not accommodate complex causality.

Davies and Nutley offer a discussion of what is a classical experimental design, the notions of research quality that define it, and how it stands at the apex of hierarchies of quality evidence operating in health.[111] That discussion is consistent with the view presented in this book that classical experimental studies have considerable value for health policy, though they need to be enriched with a broad range of other information important to understanding such things as the costs, risks, and benefits of particular policy actions. Further, without adaptation the longer time frames of experimental research may be unsuited to the needs of policy-makers. Experimental designs are most often valuable to policy when used in conjunction with other methods or in modified form to meet the needs of policy-makers. Their great value for policy-making is that when properly designed they can provide strong evidence of the outcomes of an intervention with confounding factors controlled.

The aim in research for policy may include a reflective extension of the principles of classical experimental studies to meet the needs of evidence-based policy-making.[112] 'Translational research' for health policy has often included an (admittedly conservative) emphasis on adapting features of randomized controlled trials to ensure greater external validity while retaining the scientific rigour that has been a hallmark of the experimental approach. The researcher is thus involved in making trade-offs in research design between features of research approaches aimed at external versus internal validity.[106] The challenge is to make design decisions and use measurement techniques that add to the external validity of classical experimental designs and detract as little as possible from the internal rigour of the design.

A critical area in which classical experimental studies can be adapted for policy-making contexts relates to the use of randomization. One key strategy is to work with policy-makers to develop methods of randomization that will work for them, especially if there are political constraints on randomization. This discussion can focus on the level of randomization of participant individuals that is feasible; for example, randomization by a geographic unit such as a health clinic.[55] Of course, random selection is not always feasible (or ethical) in policy contexts, so other approaches need to be used. One is repeating the experimental study in many different areas using diverse subject pools until generalization to the larger population in question becomes possible.[55] However, this can be too time-consuming and expensive and there can also be political constraints. Other solutions must be found. Fortunately, there are some useful papers about how to adapt clinical trial methodology for the needs of policy-makers and service development using cluster trials and non-randomized trials.[113] This literature offers strategies that can make a study more robust or perhaps robust enough for the nature of the decision that must be made using those data. However, valid randomization rightly remains the gold standard for avoiding confounding from unknown variables.[55]

Key practical strategy

An important paper by Tunis and colleagues offers insights into the nature of 'pragmatic clinical trials' (PCTs) which is a term given to classical experimental designs adapted to meet the needs of policy and clinical decision-makers. Some strategies offered in this paper are to

- select a range of clinically relevant interventions for comparison
- include diverse study participants in terms of population and setting characteristics
- collect data on the full range of relevant health outcomes
- base the hypothesis and the study design on information needed by decision-makers.[114]

Tunis and colleagues suggest that PCTs can yield information about risks, benefits and costs, of an intervention, not simply how and why it works for clients.[114]

Many of the methods discussed in this chapter should be considered possible adjuncts to classical experimental designs: they can be woven into the research method to enrich the findings.

When designing adaptations of classical experimental research designs to achieve greater external validity for policy-makers, it can be helpful to use a table setting out the possible range of adaptations that are being considered, as well as their strengths and weaknesses for the specific policy context being considered. This strategy, in one form or another, has been used in translational research.[106]

The resources produced by the Blair government also offer ideas for how to design a range of experimental and quasi-experimental studies in ways that are useful to public policy. Such resources concur with the view in this book that, generally speaking, high stakes complex policy-making ought not to rely solely on experimental methods.[82]

Generic features of quantitative research methods for policy-making

... the validation around the life expectancy gap of Aboriginal people is a conundrum ... depending on which one you use you either have a twenty year life expectancy gap or you have a seventeen—or in the more recent papers it's down around eleven ... And if we have three different variations in a process that gives three different age gaps then you get us an issue of credibility. The public will not understand the technical aspects of the methodology applied, what they will ask is how can a national agency come out with three different gaps in life expectancy.

(health agency CEO)

Quantitative methods share a positivist valuing of objectivity, an emphasis on deductive processes, hypothesis testing, fixed study designs and pre-determined sample sizes, and a focus on the goal of generalizing findings to a particular population. The studies involved can take the form of experimental, quasi-experimental, and observational studies: systematic reviews, meta-analyses, randomized controlled trials, cohort studies, and case-control studies. The data collection methods focus on obtaining numerical information that help understand significant variables in producing particular phenomena. The data analysis is often presented in the form of figures, graphs, tables, formulae, or theoretical models.[115]

As this book has suggested, it is sometimes argued that traditional statistical methods, especially more simplistic approaches such as significance testing, too often fail to capture the complex issues involved in delivering evidence to policy-makers.[116] However, developments in statistical techniques and associated software offer new ways of responding to the needs of policy-makers.

The discussion that follows does not attempt to cover all the technical statistical advances and tools with which highly numerate researchers for policy will be familiar or want to become familiar. Rather, the aim is to canvass some of the challenges and strategies of doing such 'numbers research' for policy-makers in ways that suggest how traditional quantitative research is being reinvented. More qualitatively trained researchers may find this discussion of interest because a critical skill in doing research for policy-makers is being able to work symbiotically with highly skilled quantitative researchers. More quantitatively trained researchers may be interested in this section for ideas on kinds of analyses that are not simply technically robust, but also speak to the policy problem in ways that help tell a policy story.

Computational modelling for health policy

The whole area of research for health policy has been undergoing great transformations as a result of computer simulations or 'computational modelling.' These tools should not be regarded as the province purely of quantitative research experts. In essence they are about flexible modelling of how different processes or mechanisms might work over time, under different conditions—the 'third way' of delivering both theoretical and applied dimensions of research.[117] A model can also be defined as an 'analytic methodology that accounts for events over time and across populations based on data drawn from primary and/or secondary sources' [118] (p.350). It can vary greatly in technical complexity.

Modelling allows researchers to answer questions policy-makers might have about, for example, how different interventions or strategies or future scenarios might work, with what costs, inputs, outputs, and outcomes. In health, modelling has been used to offer evidence for everything from public health policy to clinical practice guidelines. This area has seen recent very substantial development in the disciplines of sociology, political science, science policy, as well as business and economics.[117] Modelling for policy-making is not about finding out some conclusive set of truths as such for a policy decision-making context. It is about developing information that can be used as a decision aid for policy-making.[118] Accordingly, it often uses varied information, from meta-analysis to databases, to clinical trial data, to Delphi panel information.[119]

Forecasting for policy contexts, including forecasting the effectiveness of interventions, using quantitative methods is a key challenge of computational modelling. It involves taking data on what is known and using mathematical techniques to estimate outcomes or model what might happen in situations that do not yet exist.[1] This is a challenge because of the dynamic nature of policy contexts and the complexity of simulating or modelling the paths of policy-relevant variables.[120] A varied body of literature has developed to offer advanced statistical and mathematical applications for policy decision support, including the management of uncertainty in modelling for policy decision-making.[1, 120] It suggests that different kinds of decision support—from risk assessment to cost benefit analysis—are needed for different kinds of policy uncertainties.

The challenge of uncertainty in modelling for policy-making

Developing a decision-support model to use for health policy contexts requires a deep understanding of the nature of the uncertainty involved—not simply from a technical quantitative perspective. The table on uncertainties and certainties discussed in Chapter 2 can be used to conceptualize what is not known for the purposes of selecting probabilistic decision-modelling approaches for policy use. This kind of approach is important in modelling because what is needed is an interdisciplinary, systematic approach to decide the nature of the uncertainty at stake in a particular policy situation.[1] There needs to be a conceptual model of the nature of the decision support that is needed, which is accurately translated into the mathematical modelling process. The challenge of doing computational modelling for policy-making is about managing to deliver internal statistical and mathematical validity in ways that do not privilege that validity over the requirements for external validity for policy-makers and the community. This involves engaging with what is known and unknown in both the technical statistical and the broader policy-making sense.

Essentially, modelling uncertainty is about developing different scenarios for different health policy options which show how the outcomes of those options may be affected by specific uncertainties. The uncertainties may be technical research ones, or clinical, economic, or political uncertainties. The Blair government's guidelines for economic appraisal, *The Green Book*, includes a general introduction to uncertainty and risk management research.[72]

Deciding on what model to use for health policy-making

One key challenge for researchers is deciding what model should be used for policy decision-making. Models cannot predict the future with absolute accuracy because they can only use data from the present as a point of departure for such predictive modelling.[118] How should they be validated according to what guidelines? How can a good model be distinguished from a bad one for the purposes of health policy decision-making?

There are some published guidelines that researchers can consult for good practice in decision analytic modelling in healthcare research.[121] These suggest that the focus in assessing the quality of models for decision-making should be on the model structure, the data that are used to build the model, as well as procedures for model validation.[121] In practice, the greater the stakes in policy decision-making, the greater the verification of the model needed (where possible). The model will need to be tested against reality using independent statistics as part of verification, as well as other techniques in the technical literature.[118] However, not all models can be validated before their use, although their assumptions can receive ongoing assessment against data.[121]

Key practical strategy

Criteria used to choose a model, as well as the procedures used to validate the model, can be given in a technical report in an appendix to the main report and (sparingly) as technical footnotes. The main body of the research report should ideally include a statement to the effect that the model is a decision aid only, and concise elaboration of what are the assumptions and data on which the model is built. What is important is that the logic of the model is made as transparent as possible.[121]

Operations research

'Operations research' is an approach to research that analyses the mechanisms by which particular interventions work in the community. Frequently it involves innovative designs for taking 'street-level observations' that are then analysed with advanced mathematical techniques and computer simulation to model desirable policy. An example might be observations of needle exchange programmes and the prevention of HIV. The method has been applied to urban service development, crime and violence, drugs, and public health, at least.[122] Operations research can involve many aspects of interventions and services: health service planning and modelling, estimations of long and short-term costs, forecasting demand, estimating staffing and human resource considerations, healthcare performance modelling and any other operational areas where mathematical modelling can be applied to meet planning and policy-making needs.[123, 124] It has had particular value for innovative service development—for example, modelling aspects of a national 24-hour helpline service for the National Health Service in Britain[123] or modelling patient activity and resource use in a hospital accident and emergency department.[125]

Operations research has been adopted for use in policy-making at both the macro and micro policy level. It has been used by such organizations as the World Bank,[122] as well as at the level of developing local community interventions.[126] It also has application to clinical decision-making problems such as modelling risk during certain procedures and other clinical decision tree modelling challenges.[127] The regional agenda for health in, for example, the UK has been strongly defined by concepts of regeneration of areas of disadvantage using holistic approaches across different areas such as health, wellbeing, employment and so on. Operational research has been combined with participative approaches to gaining community involvement for designing, developing and delivering such local initiatives.[126]

Key practical strategy

Operations research can be selected wherever there is a need for 'street level' analysis involving mathematical modelling. Typically operational research involves six stages:

1 Definition of the problem and gathering of data.

2 Development of a mathematical model for representing this problem, including validation of the model.

3 Development of computer applications for solutions-finding using the model, including operating procedures implementation.

4 Testing and refinement of the model.

5 Development of areas of application of the model.

6 Implementation, including accurate translation of operating procedures, and rectifying any flaws in the approach.[128]

More sophisticated operations research offers a framework for incorporating a wide range of considerations relevant to policy decision-making: not just what actually occurs in the operation of an intervention at the grass roots level in the community, but also resource issues and trade-offs in equity and efficiency and so on.[122] The apparent disadvantage of such an approach is that it may place too great an impost on the technical expertise of community-level policy-makers. However, operations research can help challenge how policy-makers think about a problem by bringing new evidence to bear on how interventions actually operate 'on the ground' in the community. It can also offer prospective modelling of interventions and services that do not yet exist.[113] Readers wanting more detail on operations research should consult *Operations Research and Health Care: A Handbook of Methods and Applications.*[127]

Network research for health policy-making

Another interesting application of quantitative modelling lies in network research. Network research has been developed in three traditions of research: research into social networks, policy networks, and public management networks. It has involved a mixture of case studies as well as quantitative modelling techniques. It has many applications to health policy. For example, organizational networks and their role in health service delivery can be modelled in ways that explore different policy options for maximizing service delivery outcomes.[129, 130] In this method, data are collected from a wide range of sources, both qualitative and quantitative, allowing for consideration of structural and contextual features of networks operating to deliver services.

Network effectiveness can also be assessed by aggregating data collected from a wide range of sources. Analysis of qualitative and quantitative data at different levels of the organization allows consideration of the structural and contextual factors that shape network effectiveness in service delivery.[129] Such approaches can involve more advanced modelling techniques including computer simulation techniques for policy-making. These applications of quantitative modelling are particularly useful for developing policy-making about funding for, and support of, the organization of community-based health and human services.[129]

Network theory and computational modelling have many other possible applications for health policy-making.

Key practical strategy

For example, the 'Cellular Automata with Social Mirror Identity Model' (CASMIM) developed by Huang et al. allows novice researchers to create different scenarios or simulations of epidemic transmission dynamics in ways that model different combinations of responses, both preventative and suppressive.[131] The model is based on network theory or 'small world' theories used in mathematical modelling. It allows health policy-makers to consider combinations or 'suites' of policy responses such as whether the public needs to wear particular kinds of masks and what kinds of home quarantine levels might be appropriate.[131] Such simulation models are based on data about the operation of social networks in geographical regions,

Key practical strategy *(continued)*

for example, how people cluster, their long and short distance movements, and so on.[131] The approach could also be used to simulate and analyse communication problems in, for example, the functioning of human social networks for public health policy making.[131]

Using population health data for policy

Population health data exists in different forms, levels, and kinds of databases. Local databases can be used to supplement and sometimes even triangulate, data from larger national databases. Examples of useful databases are registers such as those for immunization, national disease and morbidity databases, databases on health service utilization held by government and non-government agencies, administrative health record databases held by health agencies or insurers, medical record databases held by practitioners, health service laboratory databases, and data held by linked social services including in the non-government sector.[132]

Population health data can offer 'real word' perspectives on the instrumental gain of particular relevant policies in target populations. Such studies of population health data have a particular value for health policy-makers which clinical trial data cannot provide. These data can help assess the sheer size of a health challenge, identifying affected populations, to help develop directions for policy and to provide information about the effectiveness of particular interventions for specific groups.[132]

However, such population databases are beset with problems for health policy. The validity of systems of classification for research for policy-making cannot be assumed not least because such databases are fraught with definitional problems and may be based on data constructs that do not apply in the same way, if at all, to the local policy context.[133]

Population health data should be analysed using specific research questions developed to interrogate the databases in ways that are useful to policy-makers. This may require collaboration between a skilled policy analyst and a highly skilled quantitative researcher with experience in using population health databases. However, the ability to formulate such questions will always be limited by the nature and quality of the databases themselves. When treating such databases, the researcher may want to first establish how the data were collected with an eye on establishing their validity, reliability, currency and accuracy, and so on. Considerations of data validity and credibility relevant to policy-makers, discussed earlier, should also be central to this exercise.

> ## Key practical strategy
>
> Researchers should consider networking with individuals from different organizations who perform routine data mining of such databases to audit and triangulate understandings and examine existing reports of such data. Speaking directly with those who designed the data collection items as well as those who know about their administration is of critical importance for accurate interpretation of the data.

This direct contact can be especially helpful when dealing with highly controversial data constructs. For example, in the United Kingdom there has been a great deal of debate around the collection of ethnic data on political, methodological, practical, and ethical grounds. Use of any survey data involving constructs of ethnicity and race will need to be informed by best practice in the international literature as well as an awareness that such constructions are not value free and have political consequences.[133] This means that researchers may want to liaise with the authors of those databases to develop an explanation of the deeper logic and rationale of any such constructions of ethnicity and race.[133] Triangulation, supplementation, or even substitution of parts of such databases can take place using qualitative methods such as case studies or focus group data drawn from the local community.[133]

Researchers may also want to consult studies of the pros and cons of policy-relevant tools for population health research, such as the population impact number (PIN) and disease impact number (DIN).[134] These allow comparison of the population impact of different interventions for the same or different health conditions. They offer tools for health policy-makers to take a population perspective on risk measures. Such measures have the advantage (and face the challenge) of using a complex range of peer- and non-peer reviewed data and reports, including about local contexts.[134]

Cost-effectiveness and economic evaluation

The usefulness and importance of economic evaluations are flagged here because the policy problem will often include cost effectiveness evaluation components. Engaging with contextual complexity in health policy-making also means developing economic evaluations that offer methodological rigor useful to high stakes decision-making.[135] Therefore, researchers who do not have this expertise will often either need to seek out others with technical skills in cost effectiveness research, or acquaint themselves with the relevant study designs and methods.[136]

A large body of research literature exists for students of health economics, including from public finance, about how to identify the effectiveness of health interventions.[137] This suggests a wide range of approaches to economic evaluations. Evaluating the costs of different policy options is one kind of approach, but so also is evaluating the net benefits of these options in ways that allow policy-makers to prioritize options with similar costs.[137]

Key ideas

The relationship of costs to net benefits is often important to policy decision-making.[137] Policy-makers want to know about both cost burdens and net benefits that may matter to them—not just the researcher.[81] They also want to know about the 'opportunity cost' or the true cost of an intervention in terms of the benefit foregone by funding a particular policy option rather than the second best alternative.[113]

Cost effectiveness analysis compares the differential costs gained by achieving a particular objective. Cost benefit analysis considers alternative uses of a particular resource or the opportunity cost of these different alternatives. Cost utility analysis focuses on the utility of different kinds of outcomes for those who will actually use or benefit from the policy or service.[82]

There are different models in the economic evaluation literature for calculating the relative value of different options, including more flexible ones based on an understanding of how to incorporate the objectives that matter to policy-makers.[31] These can involve the use of decision-analytic approaches synthesizing resources from many different sources to link data to outcomes relevant to policy-makers.[136] Decision analytic modelling allows models to be developed to make comparisons between treatments or interventions where the information from clinical trials is not conclusive, and where there is a need to evaluate and model what the cost effectiveness would be of implementing particular healthcare interventions.[138] In practice, operations research and economic evaluation methods often overlap, especially where operations research evaluates 'street level' economic considerations relevant to policy decision-making.

Practical tools for economic evaluations for health policy

Technical approaches to evaluating cost effectiveness are a highly contested area, including in relation to uncertainties around information for cost effectiveness.[139] The earlier discussion suggests that methods for economic evaluations in health will frequently involve more than simple metrics on cost effectiveness or benefits or their relationships. Such methods can involve synthesizes of these with multiple sources of information, both formal and informal, to deliver useful evidence for pragmatic decision-making.[57] Serious doubts have been raised about the use of simplistic calculations to find a cost-effectiveness threshold at which an intervention is not worthwhile. There are indications that simplistic cost-effectiveness ratios estimates are rarely used by decision-makers.[140] This may be because they do not take into account social contextual values such as willingness to pay for medical interventions or even competing economic priorities operating in a distinctive policy decision-making context.[141] The challenge is to develop economic evaluation information that is technically sophisticated enough to take these things into account. At the same time, researchers will also often need to include non-technical explanations of the methods of economic evaluations that allow policy-makers to see, and communicate to others, the essential value and relevance of the approaches used.[135]

A commonly used and arguably misused tool for economic evaluation is based on 'quality adjusted life-years' (QALYs). This is a way of calculating the benefit of a health intervention in terms of time in a series of quality-weighted health states, from perfect health (weighted 1.0) to dead (weighted 0.0). The quality weights for each state are multiplied by the time spent in that state, and the products are summed to obtain the total number of QALYs.[141, 142] For example, the cost of dialysis for patients with chronic renal failure has been calculated (some time ago) to be $50,000 per QALY year gained. Therefore, if, as has been the case under United States federal policy, United States citizens receive that dialysis under Medicare, the argument is that those interventions with a similar or better QALY outcome should also be offered.[141] However, reviews of literature about benchmarks derived from this tool can offer a basis for exploring why a local context may involve different numerical values. All sorts of other factors such as increases in healthcare utilization (and thus increases in costs) arising from the intervention becoming available, need to be factored into the analysis.[141] Simplistic QALY analyses need enrichment using methods that allow incorporation of social preferences for different health outcomes.

Not surprisingly, there are other proposed alternatives to QALY calculations.[142] There are voices in the health literature arguing that calculations of cost effectiveness should be based on flexible models that reflect the objectives not of policy-makers universally, but of the particular policy-makers in question.[31] Alternatives to simplistic cost-effectiveness ratios include cost-consequence analysis which is an approach to estimating the value for money of a disease intervention. In this model, the impact of the intervention is calculated using lifetime resource use and costs (such as health service use and costs and productivity losses) and health outcomes (such as disease symptoms, life expectancy and quality of life).[140] This method has the advantage that it does not give a single simplistic aggregate measure such as QALY or cost-effectiveness ratios. It does include a range of direct and indirect uses, costs, and outcomes. Accordingly, a wide range of sources of information are used, not just clinical trial data, which does present challenges of quality assurance of these different information sources. Decision-makers can use combinations of items from the model to compute composite measures, including QALY.[140]

Another tool that has been used in economic health research for policy-makers over the last three decades is programme budgeting and marginal analysis (PBMA). This approach uses the economic concepts of opportunity cost and margin to help policy decision-makers weigh up the cost and benefits of services through analysis of resource shifts.[57] Researchers can use this approach to focus not simply on efficiency, but also on equity and efficiency, at micro through to macro levels of policy decision-making.[57] The PBMA approach is essentially a priority-setting approach. It can involve using expert panels including stakeholders to rank different kinds of investments and disinvestments after consideration of relevant criteria on costs, benefits, and risks, and other business case information, as well as evidence from the wider literature, local resource projects, informal stakeholder input, and so on.[57] Such processes for making priority-setting decisions are necessary because there is not a magic tool or set of formal evidence that can answer the questions of micro or macro policy conclusively.[57]

Increasingly, decision-analytic models are being used in economic evaluations because prospective clinical studies cannot provide all the information needed.[119] The range of applications of such methods to the challenges of economic evaluations can be very broad: from financial health policy to disease management.[119] There are a number of particularly good introductory papers to decision analytic modelling in health policy research for health economics, including newer Bayesian simulation approaches sketched by Cooper et al. in a paper published in *Health Economics*.[138] The value of such approaches for policy-making is that they allow the synthesis of a broad range of information ranging from randomized controlled trials to expert opinion, into a single model that can offer a basis for considering the cost effectiveness of alternative actions.[138] However, while there are some good overviews of techniques for different approaches to cost-effectiveness analysis, including approaches that allow incorporation of social preferences for health outcomes useful to resource allocation, there is as yet a lack of consensus about measurement techniques.[142]

Cost-effectiveness analyses can also be calculated alongside clinical trials as part of a hybrid trial design. This means that the more comprehensive outcomes needed for cost-effectiveness evaluations (such as quality of life) get collected alongside the clinical trial endpoints. The two kinds of data can be mutually useful. There are some (albeit limited) models available for designing such hybrid trials such as the one developed by Ramsey, McIntosh, and Sullivan: these focus on such matters as developing approaches to hypothesis testing, sampling, and methods for collecting cost and outcome data in ways that help maximize external validity.[143]

Whatever method is chosen, researchers will want to consult the guidelines for analysis of economic evaluations that operate in different countries. These may require, for example, that particular elements of cost-consequence analysis approaches are used or that economic appraisals include specific kinds of financial information.[140] The Blair government's Treasury published guidelines on economic appraisal and evaluation for policy-makers: these offer useful insights into not only evaluation of policy and programme development, but also new or replacement capital projects, use or disposal of assets, and decisions about regulations and procurement.[72] The value of this resource as well as other toolkits for policy-makers produced by the Blair government are that they act as a general introduction to a style of economic evaluation for policy-makers that integrates economic analysis into the broader set of factors that shape policy decision-making.[72, 144] For example, and in relation to the earlier discussion on modelling uncertainty, the Treasury resource advises that economic evaluation should involve consideration of the expected values of all risks for different options, as well as a consideration of the nature and extent of uncertainty surrounding each option. It also offers suggestions for how to deal with unvalued costs and benefits that don't have a ready monetary value, through weighting such costs and benefits via community consultation. [72]

Evaluation of financial performance

Evaluation of financial performance is another important area of economic evaluation. The question of financial performance is a question that can be answered at a micro, meso, or macro level. It can involve very different questions at each of these levels from 'What did it cost to treat a patient'? to 'How do comparable health services in rural areas compare with urban centres in terms of health technology infrastructure costs?' This presents particular challenges not least because of the limited nature of data on financial performance of health services such as hospitals in, for example, the United States, United Kingdom, and Australia at least, but also the fact that when these data are available, they are often not in user friendly forms.[22, 145] This can make it difficult to construct categories for meaningful analysis and comparison of financial performance.[145] In the United States in the 1970s, diagnosis-related groups (DRGs) were used to establish standardized cost data for particular hospitals. They involved 'casemix profiles' or summaries of types of patients and relative costliness. However, the complexities of hospital funding methods meant that such evidence did not always feed directly into changes to policy.[22]

Key practical strategy

When producing analyses of financial performance for health policy-makers, researchers should consider including other kinds of information that give these data meaning. For example, data analyses of the financial performance of rural general practices is of little use unless it is included alongside other data analyses about the costs, inputs, outputs, and outcomes achieved from those health services. Thus, financial performance analyses should be considered separately, but in the wider context of other information about service and systems performance. Researchers should consult with policy-makers or their advisors to schematize the total set of information that will be required to make information on financial performance meaningful.

Researchers should consult different examples of how financial performance is measured in different systems. The case studies at the end of this chapter include a detailed analysis of performance measurement research for public hospital systems in which financial performance is integrated into analyses of other aspects of performance.

Market level research

Another area of economic research is market-level research for healthcare. Typically this research is defined by modelling of healthcare services under different market conditions and financial models, and competition modelling based on a market-driven approach to the provision of healthcare.[146] Associated with this literature are debates about what are the best approaches for measuring markets and competition in healthcare. These debates include debates about how healthcare markets should be defined and at what level they should be analyzed using what mathematical approaches, for example, for computations of market concentration.[147]

The ultimate aim of much research in healthcare market reform is often in line with corporate strategy goals, although of course such research also has a role in cost-effective public policy making contexts. This research can lie at the interface of economic and social goals, for example, as in economic research on how to manage specific aspects of healthcare markets (such as hospital ownership changes) to achieve particular social goals such as quality.[148]

There are persuasive arguments that market-level research for healthcare faces challenges that distinguish it from market-level research for other sectors,[147] although there are commonalities. The differences can arise from the different business and market structure of healthcare. The commonalities can arise from ways in which on healthcare markets behave like other markets.[146] Such research also faces multidisciplinary challenges to do with understanding the nature, preferences, and organizational behaviours of policy-makers.[146]

Key practical strategy

Market level research can benefit from supplementation with sociological approaches.[146] There are a range of possible theoretical frameworks that can be used, from organizational theory to social network theories. Social network theories in particular can help researchers better understand how inter-organizational relationships affect policy-makers preferences and how different policy options can affect healthcare organizations' bargaining. This can add an important dimension to market-level research for policy.

Comparative systems analyses

> ... but what we found in the NHS is it's very difficult, something that's worked in one place and you put it somewhere else and don't get the same effect, and I think that's sometimes because the context isn't researched in the right way. So what are the filters and factors and things that influence what actually happened?
>
> (health agency CEO)

Related to the economic evaluation literature are approaches to evaluating the performance of a system against policy goals, about which there is a growing yet still embryonic body of scholarly literature: comparative studies within national frameworks and research conducted by international health agencies such as the World Health Organization.

Evidence about the relative performance of different models in terms of policy objectives is of vital interest to policy-makers. This will be evidence based on usually quantitative measures constructed to assess the performance or results of models, systems, organizations, and programmes. However, as has been suggested, many aspects of healthcare systems cannot be very well captured by traditional quantitative approaches. A key difficulty for researchers for policy is that while half of the OECD countries have heavily invested in performance measurement systems, there is relatively little formal evaluation of these systems themselves.[86] Further, as has been noted of, for example, the UK National Health Service, the performance information within a system (not just across systems) may be asymmetrical and the objectives incompatible.[86]

In his book *Fads, Fallacies and Foolishness in Medical Care Management and Policy*, Marmor argues that the vast majority of comparative studies in health policy do not provide a sound base for lesson drawing. The reasons include the poor quality of such comparative studies: caricaturing rather than characterizing health systems; compiling comparisons that suggest different characteristics are the same and vice versa; not making modest enough claims about the lessons that may be drawn from the comparisons. He concludes that such studies need to pay better attention to specific questions to do with what features of a health system can be applied in another system under what circumstances, bearing in mind institutional and cultural factors.[149]

> . . . we often ignore or we don't spend enough time thinking about . . . if you add something into a system it will distort something else in that system.
>
> (health agency CEO)

As was suggested by Chapter 3 on reviewing the evidence, comparison of evidence relating to the performance of different systems will involve triangulating 'hard' quantitative information with 'soft' information such as information from qualitative studies or informal sources obtainable from, for example, clinician networks.[86] In the face of serious gaps in evidence, the researcher will need to use an approach that allows the different kinds of information to supplement and triangulate one another. Decisions need to be made about the kinds of measures of performance that matter. This may also involve deciding on some defined norm or standard against which the different systems or models can be compared.

Key practical strategy

For example, the researcher may develop 'league tables' of the different systems using norms derived from a range of data about past experiences of the particular system, as long as they are norms relevant to the policy-making context.[86] This may involve developing portfolios of information about different systems and subjecting them to expert scrutiny to develop measures of performance relevant to the policy-making context.

There are useful tools for ranking and comparing units of health provision against policy goals for the purposes of policy decision-making and analysis.[150] These use empirically derived sets of attributes to rank different kinds of units of health provision such as different care systems or organizations. Where the attributes are not available, or their weightings difficult to determine, the research literature can also be used to develop weighted attributes.[150] Evaluation of their utility, however, is often from the perspective of statistical internal validity, such as what to do about missing data,[150] rather than their external validity for policy-makers. Some ranking techniques can provide different rankings as an artefact of, for example, result of how missing data is managed.[150] This is not the same as those services so ranked actually being different in terms of policy goals they have reached.

Accordingly, such quantitatively derived ranking techniques for benchmarking health services need to be balanced with qualitative approaches. Qualitative approaches can help explore the underlying causes and the contextual complexities to do with why different systems perform differently. In the absence of such triangulation, such ranking techniques may be given greater importance in policy decision-making than they warrant.

The nature and uses of qualitative methods for health policy

Qualitative methods involve a focus on understanding multiple realities in which subjectivity is an accepted part of the research approach. The methodological underpinnings are inductive, with flexible design where the sample size is not always predetermined, and the goal is to identify themes that may be applicable to other contexts. Examples of qualitative approaches are grounded theory, phenomenology, ethnography and participatory action research, case study approaches, and descriptive narratives of various kinds. The data collection methods often focus on obtaining language data that help understand phenomena from a holistic perspective. The evidence available to qualitative researchers may be by way of direct observation, electronic recording, pictures, documents and so on.[151] The data analysis is often presented in the form of themes, or narratives, or theoretical models.[115]

A detailed discussion of the traditions, nature, and value of qualitative research for policy is given by Philip Davies in *What Works? Evidence Based Policy and Practice in Public Services*.[152] Readers should also consult the introductory book *Qualitative Methods and Health Policy Research* by Murphy and Dingwall.[151] The discussion that follows highlights the possibilities of qualitative research for health policy, rather than offering details of its many different applications.

Qualitative research has value because it can offer rich descriptions and explanations of complex events, perspectives and values, including that of stakeholders in a particular policy context. Qualitative research can have great value for understanding difference, such as differences between different stakeholder views, including cultural minorities. It can also be important for answering complex, open-ended questions about the nature and extent of community perceptions of the effectiveness of policy directions, or of the different political agendas held by different community stakeholders.[153]

Qualitative research can also help build abstract understandings, theories, and hypotheses useful to research for policy.[153] Policy-making requires understanding causality at multiple levels, a style of multi-level theorizing that requires more than just variable-driven approaches characterizing the less innovative quantitative research techniques.[107] This theorizing can be greatly aided with qualitative approaches.

In particular, qualitative methods can help capture the nature of practice and its organizational contexts, as Murphy and Dingwall have pointed out.[151] This can be important to understanding a particular policy problem and its solution when, for example, the policy problem relates to how health practices and organizations work from day-to-day. Thus qualitative approaches can help uncover system-level issues and solutions by capturing the dynamic nature of settings and human actions.[151]

Qualitative methods can also have value in developing understandings of how and why policy interventions have worked in particular ways in different organizations, communities, and markets.[153] Such methods are useful for answering complex evaluation questions to do with how well intervention implementation processes are working. Qualitative methods also have value for helping to decide about appropriate methods and materials for policy development and implementation. For example, focus groups can be used to help develop the content of messages and materials useful to disseminating different policy options.

A key challenge in research methods for policy is how to use information that falls outside the formal scholarly literature, such as anecdotal information which can sometimes be undervalued. Information from influential policy networks falls into this category. Qualitative research methods offer ways of capturing such anecdotal language data from policy networks, for example, using language-based analyses.

Qualitative research methods have particular value for revealing the substantive issues that lie behind policy arguments and the language used by different stakeholders in relation to a policy problem. Such language-centred approaches can be used not merely to diagnose what is really being communicated in written and spoken words, but also to expose assumptions behind those words in ways that potentially take away their political power. Researchers for policy-makers are not simply engaged in an exercise of mounting empirical evidence. They are also engaged in speaking back to political contexts shaped by the language used by many players, from policy-makers, to experts, to community members, to the media. Being able to give policy-makers a language that will reveal and neutralize the assumptions in the language that fuels policy differences can greatly add to the researcher's toolbox of effective skills. As Chapter 7 suggests, often this language of refutation is modelled in the research report, in the telling of the policy story. There are arguments about the moral and intellectual value of this kind of 'unmasking' in the policy analysis literature which has been associated with the work of Deborah Stone.[154, 155] However, it does draw on a well-established tradition of analysing the power of language to shape reality, associated with the writings of Michel Foucault.[156]

Qualitative methods can also have particular application to the challenges of policy priority-setting. Priority setting is about how to distribute resources in a context where those resources are limited and there are competing programmes and groups. It is likely to be needed at the macro, meso, or micro levels of policy-making.[157] Research for policy priority-setting can involve case studies, development of ethical frameworks using interdisciplinary research information, and 'action research' (discussed later). Essentially, research for policy priority-setting is about bringing together many different kinds of quantitative and qualitative information to ensure that resource allocation or rationing is informed by these different kinds of evidence.[157]

Of course, priority-setting is not simply about the question of how to set priorities. It is also about knowing when the priority-setting has been done well.[157] Thus narrow economic quantitative information is not sufficient, because there must be some framework for deciding values and for integrating the different kinds of knowledge. For example, one such model for priority-setting is 'Accountability for reasonableness', an ethical framework developed in the United States based on a notion of fairness in priority-setting involving four conditions: relevance, publicity, appeals, and enforcement.[157, 158] However, any such ethical frameworks will need to be carefully weighed for their relevance to a particular policy setting.

Key ideas

Without qualitative methods, policy analysis cannot be well-informed by approaches that capture the subjective and value-laden nature of much of the evidence that needs to be gathered and considered. In a sentence, qualitative methods have value in understanding the relative nature of truth in many policy contexts.[153]

There is considerable debate in different disciplines about the 'fuzziness' of much qualitative research. As its defendants have said, pointing to, for example, models for best practice in conducting interviews, there is much that can be done to design rigorous qualitative methods, suited to the nature of the inferences that are being made.[90]

In this book, the emphasis is on using qualitative and quantitative methods in a complementary manner to supplement and triangulate findings. The issue in policy-making is not which piece of evidence has the best internal validity, or generalizability and so on, but rather whether the collective weight of evidence is sufficient for a particular decision. The higher the stakes riding on a decision, the more robust the evidence required.

Qualitative approaches for health policy

Specific qualitative techniques that can be used in data collection for health policy include interviews, focus groups, Delphi techniques, and case studies. Qualitative theoretical tools can also be used for analysing texts and theory building: discourse analysis, hermeneutics, social reproduction, and many others. There are also qualitative approaches such as ethnography that offer both a theoretical tool and a method for data collection. Qualitative researchers have traditionally analysed their data using inductive methods, presenting their findings using a range of examples. Narrative approaches are often used to produce thematic discussion and analysis of language texts. The categories for analysis are often said to be deduced from the dataset after it is collected. The process of qualitative analysis may involve computer-assisted qualitative data analysis software that allows data to be loaded, coded, and sorted electronically.[151]

A description of qualitative approaches useful to health services and policy research is given by Sofaer in a helpful paper entitled 'Qualitative methods: what are they and why use them?'.[153] A more detailed introduction to qualitative methods is given in *Qualitative Methods and Health Policy Research* by Murphy and Dingwall.[151] Some such approaches are highlighted here. The lack of space devoted to standard qualitative techniques in this particular chapter relates to the fact that there are good books available on qualitative methods for health policy. In this book, special chapters have been devoted to quali-quantitative case-based approaches, community consensus-building, as well as policy story-telling, to examine in more detail approaches that are not so well covered by other readily accessible health policy monographs.

Ethnography or naturalistic enquiry involves unstructured observations and conversations, including participant observation. The researcher takes notes on the basis of these observations. A wide range of documents may also be gathered.[153] Such an approach can be helpful when there is a need to study a complex event or group of people in context. An example might be researching the culture of health service organizations with a view to policy decisions about hospital error and disclosure.

Discourse analysis is both a theoretical model of how language works and a means for structuring analysis of language texts. It includes a range of different techniques, such as those associated with the language theoretician Fairclough who has been influenced by Foucault.[159, 160] Discourse analysis can have value for understanding matters that are not 'black and white' such as the nuances of diverse community views. Discourse analysis can allow the underlying worldviews and value systems of community opinion, including those of policy-makers, to be better explained. It offers a basis for understanding the power dynamics and logic implicit in language. It can be used to add some systemacy to the analysis of language texts that traditional narrative approaches may not have. It has a wide range of applications in policy: for example, in understanding diverse community resistance to health systems reform, or analysing the language used in the media with a view to better managing communication of a policy initiative.

As Chapter 3 on reviewing the evidence suggested, document analysis to trace the evolution of a policy problem and its related policy arguments is a critical aspect of the reviewing task. Document analysis is a demanding area of researching for policy, not least because it requires sophisticated understandings of, for example, the ways in which subtexts operate, and how the same words can mean different things or vice versa over the history of evolution of a policy argument. This kind of linguistic dance and subterfuge is where discourse theory can be most valuable to the researcher for health policy, as the work of leading policy analyst Debra Stone on how metaphors operate in policy-making suggests.[155] However, discourse analysis needs to be carefully managed in reports for policy-makers to ensure that the technical detail of this approach does not overwhelm the content of the policy report and render it inaccessible to the lay reader.

Case-study research refers to a broad collection of approaches to analysing single cases or events or a process happening over time. It may involve multiple events, not always chosen randomly. Often it involves purposive sampling of sites, informants, and so on. The data collection involves more structured research questions: for example, in interviews, and structured observations of events and documents.[153] The structured analysis of documents can involve an analysis of assumptions, values, and priorities, in ways that include qualitative methods such as discourse analysis.[153] Case-study approaches can be useful when there is a need to examine and compare different kinds of models useful for progressing a particular policy option. However, in health research case study approaches have often been considered part of 'grey literature' because they lack the robustness and generalizability of random sampling methods characterizing classical experimental designs. Fortunately, in recent years there have been major developments in case study methods associated with the work of Charles Ragin and others.[161] The next chapter focuses exclusively on the work of Charles Ragin, because small-N situations present particular challenges for rigorous methods in policy-relevant research.

Interviews represent another key technique for qualitative research for health policy. This normally involves asking questions, ranging from highly structured to open-ended questions. However, interviewers may also use vignettes or short stories to help elicit responses. For example, particular client groups such as young people may respond better to a story about a young person's experiences of health services as a way of offering their views of the adequacy of health services. Interviews can be useful as a supplement to observational methods or when the latter are not feasible. However, interpreting data from them requires sophisticated rather than literal understandings of how truth as such is influenced by social and contextual constraints and unknown factors.[151] A comprehensive account of these traps of interpretation is given by Murphy and Dingwall in *Qualitative Methods and Health Policy Research*.[151]

Qualitative researchers also make frequent use of focus groups, as a variant of interview methods. This involves bringing together people who have been selected on the basis of their characteristics, for example, representatives of particular stakeholder groups. Typically there are a limited number of open-ended questions used by the researcher who is interested in capturing a rich range of perceptions emerging out of the group dynamics.[153] Focus groups can be useful in helping refine the definition of the policy question, or gathering perceptions of the validity of data collection instruments to be used with community groups, or obtaining perceptions of the ways in which the draft research report may be read by different groups. Ideally such approaches will be used in conjunction with quantitative techniques in the interests of exploring the policy problem under consideration.

How should qualitative research be designed for health policy research? The paper on how qualitative research should be judged, cited in Chapter 3 on reviewing,[92] suggests that qualitative research can be designed with three criteria in mind. These are about ensuring the synthesis of subjective meanings, the description of wider social context, as well as the incorporation of lay people's knowledge are robust, reliable, and valid.[92] In practice this also means developing and applying qualitative methods in ways that are tailored to the policy brief. An introduction to designing and implementing qualitative approaches is given in the Blair government's resources for delivering research for public policy-making.[82] Readers should also consult guidelines for assessing the quality of qualitative research published by the UK government's Cabinet Office.[94]

Key practical strategy

Researchers might also like to carefully consider the advice about how to achieve rigour in qualitative methods, particularly in relation to sampling, given by Murphy and Dingwall in *Qualitative Methods and Health Policy Research*.[151] As they argue, sampling of participants and settings, and analysis of qualitative data, can be done in principled and strategic ways in qualitative research, however rarely it may be possible to achieve statistical representativeness. Efforts to make qualitative research more rigorous can include searching for contradictory evidence, combining different methods, cross-checking findings with research participants, and offering clear accounts of the process of data collection and analysis.[151]

> I get dissatisfied when I see research findings that are based on very small numbers of respondents . . . maybe a twenty page report is written that's drawing on twenty people . . . I get frustrated with that.
>
> (health agency CEO)

Researching sustainable development for health policy

> . . . we've tended to think of the now and potential projections for the next four years. We've not taken a futuristic position in research that says 'What is this going to show us in twenty years time?'
>
> (health agency CEO)

The UK government's review of policy-making practices in that country concluded in 1999 that the pressures of electoral cycles had created 'real obstacles to long-term thinking':

> Too often policy makers react to major problems, formulate solutions, take decisions, implement them, and move on to the next set of problems without being able to take the long-term view the White Paper envisages. (u.p.)[44]

However, sustainable development is a highly contested concept in the political and scientific domains.[162] This is partly because the concept of sustainability is multi-faceted and ambiguous. It relates to the extent to which the environment or context of an intervention is conducive to its long-term feasibility and survival. It is a concept that includes a broad range of factors such as community health service infrastructure that make a particular policy option viable in the long term. The length of the term of sustainability required may be defined by policy-makers as up to and including the next election. If that is a very short time away, the real long-term sustainability of the policy option may be less important to the policy-maker. Researchers may have fidelity to much longer timeframes in their notions of sustainability, for ethical reasons to do with their accountability to local communities.

The sustainability of health policy is a much neglected area, both theoretically and practically, in a context where the literature on sustainability places much more emphasis on notions of sustainable development of communities as such. However, analysis of the sustainability of health policy options is a real world necessity for policy-makers.

Key ideas

At the simplest level, what policy-makers need to know about sustainability is whether a particular policy option will be sustained in a particular community or region over the time of interest. This may be related to issues to do with the sustainable financing of the intervention over the long-term—which is seen in many countries as one of the most pressing issues in health reform.[163] To answer that question even in a preliminary form, there needs to be evidence of the match between the resource requirements of the option for its sustainability and the resources available in a community for meeting those requirements.

Quantitative models can offer approaches for the analysis of future sustainability, as the earlier discussion on modelling suggests. That is, quantitative models can offer demographic and social accounting for futures analysis. However, qualitative methods can also be used in conjunction with quantitative analysis to offer ways of synthesising language data that otherwise could not be included in such future analysis.[164] Qualitative methods can be used to process expert opinions in ways that use interpretative structural modelling and scenario writing.[164]

There is no single model for developing research into sustainability of policy. However, conceptual modelling of resources (more broadly understood) can be used as a point of departure for evaluating the sustainability of particular health policy options in a specific community or region, including through quantitative futures modelling.[162] The conceptual model given subsequently here can be adapted to help think through research methods for advising policy-makers whether a policy option is sustainable i.e. the match between what resources are required for that policy option to be sustainable and what resources are available in a community. Understandings of this match will ideally come not only from literature reviews, but also from consultations with policy-makers, experts, and the community members themselves. The conceptual model of resources for evaluating sustainability developed by Grosskurth and Rotmans, who build on approaches used by the World Bank, can be used as a point of departure for first understanding the broad domains under which resources may be grouped (social, environmental, and economic) before defining the particular resources of interest. There can then be further definition of the characteristics of those existing resources that are already held or need to be held in the communities of interest. This further definition should involve not simply characteristics to do with the amounts of those resources, but also their quality, function and spatial characteristics.[162]

For example, a local hospital in a rural community can be understood in terms of quantity measures such as service utilization, quality issues to do with its efficiency, the function of the service, as well as spatial characteristics to do with the material and built infrastructure, and so on. Of course, there are more complex human resource considerations such as the extent to which that health service has, over time, developed collaborative ways of working and sharing with other health and community services. These can also affect how 'wealthy' that community is in more intangible ways. If the local hospital doesn't have the necessary level of this 'social capital', a policy intervention that requires this kind of social resource may not work without particular kinds of workforce development. Research designs for sustainability will often need to regard these characteristics as interacting, when the whole set of relevant resource domains must be considered.

Once the characteristics of interest for sustainability have been described, indicators will need to be developed from them. Indicators are used to design research approaches capable of finding out more about the performance of the characteristics of interest. Figure 4.1 offers a simplification of the Grosskurth and Rotman conceptual model, adapted here for the purposes of health policy research along the single dimension of 'social capital' which can include institutional capital such as a hospital.[162] Its value is as a tool for giving researchers ways of thinking about what resources a policy option requires, which can be used to design systematic approaches to collecting evidence about its sustainability. The diagram can also be used to identify ambiguities that are part and parcel of the complex concept of sustainability

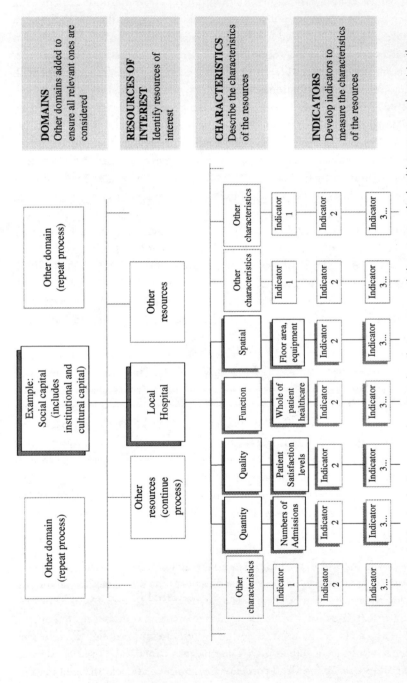

Fig. 4.1 A conceptual model for developing research approaches that measure existing community health resources relevant to the sustainability of policy options.

in ways that can make clearer what needs to happen to make an intervention sustainable.

To be useful to policy decision-making, the conceptual model outlined in Figure 4.1 needs to be implemented in ways that allow data to be collected about the time factors that shape sustainability: the longevity of resources in a community, the timeframes for intervention implementation, the political terms that are meaningful to policy-makers, and so on. This conceptual model can also be used as a point of departure for evaluating the sustainability of the policy option after its implementation, when the decision point is about whether it should be continued.

Recommended reading

Government Chief Social Researcher's Office. Magenta Book: Guidance Notes on Policy Evaluation. 1997 [online]. Cabinet Office. Available at: http://www.nationalschool.gov. uk/policyhub/magenta_book/index.asp. Accessed 21 May, 2008.

Case studies in designing research methods for health policy

Case study: Canada, climate change, and methodologies for dealing with uncertainty in health policy-making

Human Health in a Changing Climate: A Canadian Assessment of Vulnerabilities and Adaptive Capacity[165] is a major book-length study published in 2008 by the Canadian government. It represents the first study of its kind in Canada, offering an assessment of how climate change may affect the health of Canadians. It aimed to help policy-making at the federal, provincial, territorial, and municipal government levels in public health, healthcare delivery, emergency management, and community social services. That is, the report aimed to help these Canadian policy-makers better target their resources, policies, and programmes in a climate changing world. The study involved a vast amount of evidence, including existing models of adaptive capacity, to provide an analysis of how a changing climate may affect Canadians. The report identified increased health risks arising from extreme weather events including extreme heat particularly for already vulnerable communities, changes in air quality (for example from smog, wildfires, and pollen production), and infectious diseases in regions where they were previously rare or exotic. It suggested that these changes will interact with other changes, such as in demography and infrastructure, to present Canadians with new challenges. The report identified gaps in public health and emergency management that may well act to prevent effective adaptation to climate change. It advocated an approach to adaptation that was about tailor-making responses to meet the different needs of diverse vulnerable groups.

Understanding the effects of climate change on health involves the methodological challenge of deciphering different pathways for those effects (both direct and indirect) as well as the different timings for these effects. Climate change research often involves the added challenge of dealing with a sequence of events or conditions. The need to offer information about health costs and benefits further compounded these methodological challenges.

In the Canadian report, the following strategies were used to help meet these methodological strategies:

◆ use of literature scans and consultative mechanisms to help determine the structure and scope of the study

◆ use of literature reviews of scholarly and 'grey literature', including applied policy literature, to identify what is known and unknown in the field; this included reviews of documentation of indigenous knowledge and experience of climate change

◆ use of two regional studies (of the province of Quebec and Canada's North) to offer a baseline for extrapolating the relationship between climate change and health i.e. the ways in which multiple factors may interact in any one region and the adaptive capacities of that region in the face of these confounding health issues

◆ use of climate change modelling and scenario-building using multi-factoral data to simulate and predict climates

◆ use of epidemiological data and ecological studies conducted in Canada; this included ecologically oriented epidemiology studies focussing on relationships between the health of particular populations and the occurrence of particular health conditions

◆ use of stakeholder consultations, with government, non-government, research and private agencies; this included a stakeholder reference group, expert workshops, and consultations at local and regional levels to collect observations of climate change and its effects; the stakeholder consultations also helped refine understandings of Canadian policy-makers' needs in ways that reshaped the study

◆ use of experts to synthesize information and make judgements about it in key informant interviews.

Each of these methods carried its own limitations that were documented in the study. For example, literature reviews of the scholarly research faced the difficulty that many such studies have limited generalizability to the specific challenges faced by Canada's populations and regions. For some areas, such as the study of food security, there was little methodological precedence in the scholarly literature. The climate change literature also had not yet developed sufficient methodological sophistication for the sort of health vulnerability assessment that the Canadian study required. Further, climate change modelling and scenario-building around, for example, air quality issues, were in this Canadian study found to be limited by missing data and uncertainties around future conditions, including human behaviour. Epidemiological studies were expensive and time-consuming and also required a level of understanding of system dynamics that could not easily draw on existing approaches in the epidemiological literature. The Canadian study also suggests the limitations of big-N epidemiological data for complex health policy making that must involve an assessment of climate change issues for smaller vulnerable populations. Stakeholder consultations using qualitative methods were found to present the classic challenges of such methods (reliability and generalizability) with an added nuance: how stakeholders understood climate change shaped the nature of the observations they provided. Expert judgment, however, carried another kind of subjectivity (discipline bias) that was also difficult to assess.

Some of the aforementioned points suggest the major challenge in this study: the problem of uncertainty. This arose from gaps in the scientific knowledge, as well as uncertainties arising from the research methods and research outputs. Another element of uncertainty was introduced by the lack of sophisticated theories for understanding system dynamics as they operate at the different local to national levels to shape how individuals, communities, and agencies such as governments adapt to climate change. However, the study aimed to add value to policy-making by identifying the different kinds of 'unknowns', such as the uncertainties around the magnitude of particular changes and pressures on health services, and the degree of vulnerability of particular populations. The report suggests that identifying what is unknown can be most useful to policy-makers in assessing risk.

The value of the study can also be described in terms of how it synthesized information from different sources and disciplines—information about for example, regional population health data with international studies of climate change with applied policy literature—in ways that had not previously been done before for Canada. The local and particular challenges of climate change could thus be addressed in a manner that had some rigour.

Case study: Designing hospital performance evaluations for policy—Australia's *The State of Our Public Hospitals Report 2008*

The State of Our Public Hospitals Report 2008[166] suggests how Australia is meeting the challenges of developing policy-relevant performance measurement research evidence for its free public hospital system. The report is part of a series produced by the Australian government each year since 2004, providing an overview of not only the current state of Australian hospitals, but also information about a particular focus area such as rural and remote Australia, or older citizens. In 2008 the focus area was indigenous Australians.

The report gives performance information for Australian hospitals at the state, territory, and national levels. The main body of the report presents short commentary in laypersons' language illustrated with simple tables, bar charts, and pie graphs. These are arranged under headings in the form of questions such as 'What services do the hospitals provide?' and 'How long did patients stay in hospitals?' and 'What did it cost to treat a patient?' Technical elaboration is provided by way of a reference guide offering hyperlinks to key areas within the main report. These give further information such as selection criteria, source, and related other figures for data provided in the main report.

The report drew on a range of published sources such as reports from the Australian Government Treasury and the Australian Institute of Health and Welfare, as well as specific state and territory government information.

The report was informed by the data dictionary developed by the Australian Institute of Health and Welfare, however, work still needed to be done developing robust definitions for data analysis. For example, there was a need to refine what the term 'patient' excludes and includes in a context in which many patients in the public hospital system are privately funded.

Another challenge lay in the fact that Australian states and territories report their hospital level data differently. For example, some states do not provide performance information from individual hospitals on particular key areas such as safety and quality of care, though all can report data on other key areas such as elective surgery.

The study did not offer a way of evaluating whether the outcomes reported were acceptable (although admittedly, this would have taken the report beyond its brief). For example, it points out that 'Around 70% of patients at emergency departments were seen within clinically recommended times in 2006–07' (p. 46) without offering a clinical or value-based framework or performance benchmark that could be used to evaluate whether policy-makers should consider this percentage to be acceptable. However, the presentation of the special section on indigenous health does offer frequent comparison of indigenous health data with non-indigenous health data.

The results of *The State of Our Public Hospitals Report 2008* were used to illustrate and showcase the importance of the Rudd government's key hospital reforms which aimed to redress over a decade of neglect of the hospital system by the Howard government: extra funding for reducing elective surgery waiting times, establishment of an agency to drive large-scale hospital reforms, investment in family practice 'super clinics', and investments in hospital infrastructure and health workforce reform. It could be argued that while the main policy implications of the report lie in its use to improve hospital performance, the focus on aggregating data means it offers 'broad brush' policy implications for Australian states, at best.

Case study: Complex causality in the United States' National Evaluation of the State Children's Health Insurance Programme: A Decade of Expanding Coverage and Improving Access

In line with a Congressional mandate, this report evaluated the operation of a federal programme in the United States: The State Children's Health Insurance Programme (SCHIP).[167] The SCHIP essentially expanded public healthcare cover to low income children who were uninsured. What Congress wanted to know was how effective was the intervention. Evaluations of complex real world interventions such as SCHIP offer an interesting opportunity to reflect on a critical challenge of designing methods for health policy: how to capture complex causality in ways that allow policy-makers to be confident that they understand more precisely why an intervention was effective or not and what that means for future decision-making.

The research methods used in this report were framed by hypotheses of interest to the policy-making issues at hand. These were hypotheses that SCHIP would improve access to care in particular defined ways, such as realized access (to do with service utilization) and perceived access (to do with the perceived adequacy of services). Quantitative, qualitative, as well as case study approaches were used, drawing on multiple data sources.

The quantitative approaches involved analyses of, for example, population data on trends in the number and rate of uninsured children, as well as trends in enrolment and retention in the programme. The qualitative methods included synthesis of a diverse range of scholarly and applied or literature on issues such as access to care under the intervention. Qualitative data collection exercises were also used to study complex phenomena such as the nature of state outreach efforts to enrol low-income children in the intervention. The case studies involved analyses of how the programme was conducted in eight states in a context in which states were expected to tailor their implementation of the programme to their unique contexts.

The report combines qualitative and quantitative approaches to engage with complex causality important to policy decision-making. For example, policy-makers needed to know how effective were the different outreach methods used to increase enrolments of children in the intervention. This challenge was met to some extent by using quantitative methods to identify phenomena such as increases or spikes in enrolment in the programme at the state and local levels with qualitative methods identifying what kinds of outreach efforts were being used by states to try to increase these enrolments. Thus, associations could be found between spikes in enrolments and particular outreach efforts.

Another kind of challenge to do with complex causality related in this report to the issue of how to understand variation across the different states in retention rates of children in the intervention that was expected to increase public health coverage. It was in the nature of the intervention that the conditions under which each of the states implemented it were not the same. This challenge was partly met, for example, by examining trends in the continuity of public health coverage and relationships between these trends and changes in state administrative policies. However, the report acknowledges that reasons for variations in children's access to care across states remained unclear. The lack of consistent methods for measuring SCHIP performance across the states also played a part in confounding the data.

The methodological challenges to do with understanding complex causality in this report were also about what kinds of values should be used to define constructs for measuring effects. For example, the intervention was not intended to be considered effective where it acted to encourage families to drop out of their existing private healthcare cover for public health cover, and in fact states initiated disincentives to prevent this from happening. However, this 'substitution' of private healthcare cover for the intervention SCHIP is a complex construct and exceedingly difficult to measure. Clearly, it depends on how substitution is defined using what values. Under what circumstances is such substitution acceptable? The evaluators in this report used three different kinds of studies to examine this issue: population-based data and modelling (which relied on a definition of substitution as any decline in private coverage within the population of low-income children who were eligible for SCHIP, regardless of the reason), as well as enrolee- and applicant-based studies (which took into account particular reasons for the loss of coverage to do with, for example, the unaffordability of coverage). By using these different data sources and methods the evaluators were then able to offer different statistics about the extent of substitution. These illuminated the importance of policy-makers deciding on the values they wanted to bring to the issue of substitution.

This report is generally characterized by the analysis of multiple studies often at the state or local level to provide an overall national picture. This involved development of criteria for inclusion and exclusion of such studies. The inclusion and exclusion criteria related to not simply the quality of the studies but also the extent to which they were useable for the policy-relevant research framework. For example, studies on access to care were included if they evaluated at least one measure of the policy-relevant definitions of access used by the evaluators.

By allowing for complex causality, the report does more than offer figures about whether the number and rate of uninsured low-income children had fallen in the period under study. It also shows whether and in what ways the intervention contributed to this reduction. More than that, the data were extrapolated in the report to quantify what would have happened to the uninsured number and rate of low income children if the intervention SCHIP had not existed. Analyses of, for example, sub-group data also allowed consideration of which groups did and did not benefit the most from the intervention, in ways that aimed to help future decision-making.

With this emphasis on trying to understand complex causality, the report was able to offer implications for ongoing measurement of programme performance (such as in relation to consistency of data across states), implications for future research (such as linking programme outcomes to improved health outcomes, not just healthcare access), as well as implications for policy-makers reauthorizing SCHIP (for example, ideally by standardizing some components while still allowing state flexibility).[167]

Although SCHIP gained widespread bipartisan support, the Bush administration vetoed the legislation necessary for its reauthorization.

Analysing population health data: The World Health Organization's use of disability-adjusted life years (DALYs)

In 2008 WHO published its assessment of the global burden of disease,[168] offering a comprehensive comparison of deaths, disease, and injuries across countries, as well as projections to the year 2030. The study can be considered part of WHO's mandated role to produce and disseminate health information. Not only the causes of death but also the actual loss of years of good health are measured using the concept of 'disability-adjusted life years' (DALYs).

One DALY in this report is one lost year of a healthy life. The measurement of DALYs involves calculating the sum of

♦ years of life lost arising from premature mortality (YLL)

and

♦ years of healthy life lost through living in less that full health due to disease and injury (YLD).

As the report outlines, the concept of YLL involves the number of deaths at each age multiplied by a global life expectancy for each age. The YLD for a specified cause in a specified time period involves calculating the number of incident cases in a period by the average disease duration by the weight factor. The weight factor gives the severity of the disease from 0 (which is described as perfect health) to 1 (death).[168] Thus, DALYs can be used to compare the burden of disease causing early death but little disability, with diseases that do not cause death but do cause disability. Using this concept in comparative regional analyses the report suggests that, for example, DALYs are at least twice as high in Africa than in any other region. The report also uses the concept of DALYs to provide a breakdown of this concept by disease categories and regions. For example, it concludes that unipolar depression is a leading cause of the burden of disease in the WHO regions of the Americas, Europe and the Western Pacific. It identified the high burden of disease (almost 45% of the adult disease burden) that is due to non-communicable diseases (NCDs) in low and middle-income countries.

The concept of DALYs is used to offer projections of the burden of disease in 2030. For example, unipolar depressive disorders, ischaemic heart disease and road traffic accidents are projected to be the three leading causes of DALYs in 2030. The DALY projections also suggest that HIV/AIDS will drop from being the fifth leading cause of DALYs in 2004 to the ninth leading cause in 2030. Conditions that are expected to substantially decline include lower respiratory infections, perinatal conditions, and diarrhoeal disease. Conditions that are expected to increase in importance include diabetes mellitus, road traffic accidents, chronic obstructive pulmonary disease, hearing loss, and refractive errors.

The methods used in the WHO 2008 global burden of disease study include a number of issues to do with uncertainty arising from substantial data gaps and shortcomings. These are most notable for regions with limited death registration data. This means that the information provided is useful if used to make judgements based on broad relativities, rather than finely grained decisions. Thus, the report suggests how use of DALYs in policy decision-making is about matching the nature of the method to the nature of the decision that must be made.

Chapter 5

Case-based approaches
for health policy[1]

Overview

In health and other disciplines there has been some questioning of the quali-quantitative polemic characterizing so much research practice in the last few decades. This chapter aims to suggest that the choices available to researchers for health policy are no longer about big quantitative studies of aggregated datasets versus small-N qualitative 'narrative' studies that rely on 'discourse and persuasion'.[169] It explores how Charles Ragin's writings can be used to better understand context in a hypothetical small-N community health prevention study.

The rise and rise of case-based, Quali-Quantitative Analysis

The last chapter laid the basis for understanding how debates about the relevance of research evidence are linked to the rise of case-based, Quali-Quantitative Analysis (QQA). Across multiple disciplines, QQA ostensibly arises from dissatisfactions with simplistic, variable-driven statistical methods that rely on linear, unidirectional assumptions and lack authenticity for the true diversity of human action in context.[170] Increasingly, researchers are being confronted with the

---

[1] This chapter draws on a previous publication by the author: Bell, E, Hall, R. 'Dead in the water': Is rural violent crime prevention floating face-down because criminology can't handle context?, 2007, *Crime Prevention & Community Safety* 9 (4):doi:10.1057/palgrave. cpcs.8150051, reproduced with permission of Palgrave Macmillan in *Research for Health Policy*. Readers interested in exploring research methods for community-level interventions, which can be adapted for health, might like to consult this leading journal.

demand to engage with a definition of context as 'complex webs of multiple dynamically interactive, contingent "social" relations that both constrain and facilitate the reflexive actions of research subjects'[170] (p. 462). Case-based analysis is seen as a kind of answer to the problem of how to keep the contextual integrity of cases.

At the same time, it does not appear that the rise of case-based analysis is some restatement of the divide between scientific rationalist empiricism associated with quantitative methods dominant in the sciences, and more 'interpretative' traditions associated with qualitative methods in the social sciences and humanities. Rather, case-based analysis grows out of a desire to mend the fence; a growing conviction held by many researchers that research theory and practice suffers from a serious micro–macro disconnect or a failure to adequately represent the individual-situational-community dynamics of research subjects.[171] Across many disciplines there is now a search for methods that combine 'nominal, ordinal, and narrative strategies' to capture causal complexity.[172] If large-N methods have been in the ascendancy for some decades, there are signs that case-based analysis may bring a reinvigoration not just of small-N studies, but also efforts to extend large-N methodologies.

It is too early to tell if the growing phenomenon of case-based analysis will be judged historically to have better delivered on the sometimes elusive goal of relevance to policy and practice. What is certain is that the primary methodological innovation is coming from sociology and political science and from questions about how mathematics can be better used for theory construction and empirical social research.[173] Equally certain is that the rise and rise of case-based QQA is rendering the old polemic between qualitative and quantitative research traditions passé as a new generation of researchers brings skills across both traditions, and multidisciplinary content knowledge, to the task of understanding contextual complexity.[174]

This chapter explores the work of leading case-based analyst Charles Ragin. However, Ragin is not the only case-based QQA methodologist useful to researchers for health policy. For other models, readers might like to consult Pawson and Tilley,[175] as well as George and Bennett in relation to developing 'process evaluation' methodologies and 'process tracing'.[174] Like Ragin, George and Bennett use case-based comparative analytic procedures to develop contingent generalizations. However, George and Bennett place greater emphasis on tracing sequential processes within a particular historical case,[174] while Ragin places greater emphasis on summarizing causes and outcomes for a group of cases.[161]

Key ideas

This chapter focuses on Ragin because his work offers by far the most well-developed body of writing about case-based approaches. It is recommended to readers not simply as an alternative approach to small-N research, but as one of the most sustained and persuasive critiques of the social relevance of traditional quantitative research methods to emerge out of the last century.

Ragin's method can be found in over 250 applications across multiple disciplines. However, it is relatively under-referenced in methodologically conservative disciplines such as those in health. This is so even though there are considerable pressures for methodological innovations that engage with bio-psycho-social approaches now informing policy and practice, in ways that extend traditional classical experimental approaches. A few preliminary analyses have been published about the relevance of Ragin's work to health by Ragin himself.[176, 177] The author has also published papers on Ragin's work in relation to the evidence needs of holistic health practice,[178] designing services for adolescents with substance abuse issues,[179] and the management of hospital error.[180]

QQA—terms of description

A quiet global revolution in research methodology began with the publication of Charles Ragin's much praised book *The Comparative Method* (1987).[181] Subsequently, this method of comparative case-based analysis was elaborated by Ragin and his colleagues.[161, 176, 181–184] most powerfully and fully in the 2000 monograph *Fuzzy-set Social Science*.[161] Ragin and his colleagues have also developed software to support applications of the QQA method.[185]

There is space in this chapter only for the simplest of summaries of this large and complex body of writing. Readers should also be aware that a number of variations of Ragin's method have been developed and are outlined, along with discussion of issues such as generalizability and reliability, in the recent textbook *Configurational Comparative Methods: Qualitative Comparative Analysis (QCA) and Related Techniques*.[186] The description in this chapter follows Ragin's common description of implementation of his method taking place in stages, a description variously adapted by the author for different discipline specialities.[178–180, 187]

Key ideas

In this chapter this explanation has been modified to offer a sketch of a hypothetical community health prevention project using QQA, focussing on the value of such an approach for micro-policy development i.e. policy at the local community or provincial town level. This is broad and conceptual rather than focussed on the fine detail of the method, in line with the aim of this book: to highlight possibilities for adding value to research for health policy. It is hoped that this chapter will stimulate greater awareness of the potential of Ragin's methods for health policy decision-making, including at the micro-policy level of community health prevention and intervention.

The term 'Quali-Quantitative Analysis' is used here—with apologies to Ragin—in preference to the more common term 'Qualitative Comparative Analysis' because it suggests that the method combines both qualitative and quantitative approaches as part of a transdisciplinary approach. The author's experience using the term 'Qualitative Comparative Analysis' in some health research contexts suggested how difficult it can be to convey the true nature of Ragin's approach in contexts where qualitative research has been 'convicted and hung' (admittedly sometimes with a fair trial). The term 'Quali-Quantitative Analysis' is derived from the title of a book exploring the method by a Belgium-based group: *L'Analyse Quali-Quantitative Comparée (AQQC-QCA)*.[188]

The term 'transdisciplinary' suggests the ways in which this approach is not attached to any particular disciplinary knowledge. It is a method but not a methodology nor is it attached to a discipline as such. The same cannot be said of many methods which are attached to methodologies that are in turn linked (often historically rather than in a deterministic sense) to disciplines: for example, certain qualitative practices of interpreting texts ('deconstruction') are linked to a methodology (theorizations of method) called 'discourse theory' which in turn are historically linked to the discipline of English.[189–191] The methods associated with QQA are not value-free, but they are easily translated across mathematics, sciences, humanities, and social sciences disciplines. In this sense the term 'transdisciplinary' is a legitimate but not necessarily exclusive claim for QQA.

QQA in essence

Whatever else it is, QQA is a small-N method. This is because QQA considers cases as configurations, or strings of attributes, to explore their similarities and differences. Ragin argues that the complexity and diversity of context only really becomes apparent when cases-as-configurations are the unit of analysis.[161] Yet, as will be suggested by the hypothetical scenario that follows, the approach also allows scope for systematically developing the findings of a local case-based study with reference to the larger body of evidence from the health literature.

QQA can be used with both qualitative and quantitative data, or either, from clinical procedural documents to Likert scale data about patient perceptions. In this quali-quantitative approach, the nature of the data collected does not drive the method of data analysis. What matters is that the data collected allow the researcher to make good decisions about the presence or absence of the case characteristics that are of interest, as part of a systematic approach to case-based comparisons.

Another distinguishing feature of QQA is the form of the research output it produces. Qualitative analyses produce narrative analyses. Quantitative analyses produce graphs and figures and other related numerical output. However, QQA produces a kind of summary of cases considered as configurations in the form of abbreviated combinatorial statements of causes occurring with outcomes. These 'logical equations' offer summaries of 'set-theoretic relationships'.[161, 192, 193]

Key ideas

Health policy-makers often make combinatorial decisions by asking 'Which combination of which elements of different models will work best to deliver which outcomes in this particular policy context?' Similarly, Ragin's method delivers research output in the form of combinatorial statements that help answer the question 'Which combination of which elements of cases are the conditions for which outcomes in this particular small-N context?'

A hypothetical micro-policy scenario in falls prevention

There would be four basic stages in a QQA-based, small-N community health prevention research effort. The kind of scenario involved might relate to developing holistic approaches to community falls prevention initiatives for older patients. Imagine that a researcher in a government policy unit for healthy ageing has been directed to work with a group of community stakeholders, such as health and allied health practitioners, government policy officers from different departments, health consumer advocates, and others trying to make a difference to this multi-service, multidisciplinary challenge.

Falls prevention offers a good opportunity to explore holistic health policy challenges precisely because it involves developing 'whole-of-systems' policy approaches. By some estimates, falls affect about 30% of community-living persons over the age of 65 years. Around 20% of these may require medical treatment. The general consensus in the falls literature is that falls prevention and intervention require a 'whole-of-patient' approach that engages with the wider set of complex interacting bio-psycho-social patient risk factors.[194] For example, an effective approach to falls prevention may include 'holistic' or alternative/complementary therapies (such as tai chi exercise programmes), as well as attention to the patient's environment (such as installing bathroom hand rails), and behaviours (correcting walking shoes). Best practice suggests the value of multidisciplinary team case management that includes doctors, nurses, osteopaths, podiatrists, nutritionists, community healthcare workers, exercise specialists, and so on, who can work together to address heterogeneous risk profiles.[195–203] However, whole-of-patient approaches to falls prevention remains more a best practice ideal in the literature than a reality.[204] This presents particular challenges to government health policy-makers wanting the input of their communities to make good decisions about community falls prevention initiatives in ways that will facilitate bio-psycho-social approaches to falls prevention. Education programmes have had little success because what is needed is change to the approaches taken at the 'grass roots' level of community health practice.[205]

In this hypothetical scenario, a team of community stakeholder representatives of professional and patient groups has been assembled to act as a reference group for the government policy research officer who wants to develop a community-based approach to falls prevention. It is intended that the researcher use this reference group to develop data collection methods that will be implemented by health practitioners (ideally nurses or doctors) in the three family medical practices in the town that lies at the centre of the rural community under study. The project is intended to be a basis for deciding what elements of which falls prevention strategies are needed to tailor-make the best possible local community response. An overview of the stages involved in a QQA-based approach and the related research outcomes are given below.

Stage one: tabulating and summarising cases-as-configurations

The first stage of a QQA-based study would involve tabulating and summarizing configurational information about cases.

Ideally, a broad range of qualitative and quantitative data will be used about individual (bio-psycho-behavioural), situational (environmental), and community (service) characteristics of interest in falls prevention.

The team would work together to create 'property spaces' defining the characteristics of interest. These characteristics will be the basis of the data collection of actual falls prevention cases, allowing comparisons of cases considered as configurations. Characteristics of cases (patients) in a falls prevention community study may include:

- individual biological characteristics: for example, risk factor scores using formal clinical assessment in relation to known risk factors (e.g. age, vision, sensation, strength, and balance)

- situational characteristics that may be causally related such as being widowed and living alone

- behavioural characteristics such as shoe type worn

- community service characteristics as they relate to the individual such as history of community healthcare visits

- characteristics to do with the nature of the falls outcomes for that individual: number and nature (severity) of falls.

This set of characteristics of interest can be defined in a preliminary fashion with reference to

- the international literature on causes of falls, including clinical falls risk assessment tools

- observations of such characteristics made by community stakeholder reference group members.

There will be scope to add to or modify the property spaces once the data proper from the family practices participating in the study are considered.

When the actual data collection is being done, the community research team would ask health practitioners (nurses or doctors) to fill in a 'truth table' that allows cross-tabulation of the characteristics of possibly at-risk patients in terms of the presence or absence of these characteristics for each case or patient. If the team were using later 'fuzzy set' versions of Ragin's method, the 'truth table' would involve tabulating degrees of membership of cases to the defined attributes.[193] Once the cases are tabulated by nurse practitioners, the researcher would then 'minimize' the information in the 'truth table' to obtain a number of shorthand expressions of the occurrence of configurations. These shorthand expressions represent 'logical equations' for a particular kind of falls outcome. In the community falls prevention project envisaged in this hypothetical, there will be different kinds of falls depending on their severity i.e. different kinds of outcomes. Each of these may involve similar or quite different causal conditions. Thus different falls outcomes (knee fracture, ankle sprain, hip fracture) may have similar or quite different kinds of 'logical equations'. The same falls outcome (hip fracture) may also have different logical equations.[(182)]

In summary, this first stage would produce a set of 'logical equations' providing summaries of falls-cases-as-configurations in that particular community: what combinations of bio-psycho-social or individual-situational-community conditions are suggested by the different falls cases seen in the family practices.

The aforementioned description suggests another advantage of such an approach. In comparison to statistical methods which health practitioners and community stakeholders can sometimes feel occur in a 'black box', the QQA method allows for iterative, consensual processes of compiling the truth table and minimizing the case-based information into logical equations. A researcher skilled in the techniques would certainly need to guide the process. However, the QQA method appears particularly amenable to efforts to build in external practitioner and community validity—not simply internal statistical validity— through participative methods for identifying and analysing characteristics of interest at this stage. This is an important strategy for meeting the challenges of capturing local context.

Stage two: tests of 'necessity' and 'sufficiency'

The second stage would involve doing tests of 'necessity' and 'sufficiency' of possible causal conditions as they relate to the whole set of factors relevant to falls prevention.

'Necessity' and 'sufficiency' are two terms that are important in QQA: a cause is necessary if all instances of the outcome occur with the cause, and a cause is sufficient if all instances of the cause occur with the outcome. If the community research team were using the later 'fuzzy set' version of QQA, they would be using probabilistic criteria underpinned by Bayesian probability theory.[(161)] Again, the validity of these criteria would be strengthened through iteration and consensus-seeking that involves not simply the views of the practitioner and patient stakeholders on the team, but also the body of falls prevention research found by the researcher.

The outcome of this second stage in a QQA-based falls prevention study would be information about which conditions, as they relate to the holistic set of factors implicated in falls, are necessary for particular kinds of falls outcomes, and which are sufficient.

In this way the method has the potential to help make the general and theoretical speak to the local and particular as part of developing classifications of falls (and other such holistic health challenges), and their necessary and sufficient conditions. As such, QQA opens up possibilities for better understandings of holistic health challenges in small communities, and more authentic small-*N* community-based health prevention studies.

The box below offers a very simplified example of what some logical equations and their necessary and sufficient conditions might be in this hypothetical study. In practice there will be more complex and more numerous equations. In fact, much of the value of Ragin's method lies in how it offers not so much a single causal explanation, as can be the case with traditional statistical approaches, but rather a set of summary statements that suggest different causal possibilities.

Example: Logical equations, necessary and sufficient conditions, and policy-making

In a small-*N* study of falls prevention in community-dwelling older patients attending three family practices in a town, a QQA study might produce a number of abbreviated summaries of conditions associated with particular outcomes. A number of cases (say, 65) might be summarized in a way that suggested certain conditions for a serious fall with a hip fracture (SF): no history of healthcare home visits (NHV); poor coordination and balance PCB; wearing high heels (WHH); being widowed and living alone (WLA).

NHV _ SF

NHV · PCB _ SF

NHV + PCB _ SF

NHV · PCB + WLA · WHH _ SF

The mid-level dot is used to indicate logical *and* and the addition sign indicates logical *or*. The first equation suggests that in all cases of serious falls there was no history of heath care home visits. That is, all serious falls were preceded by a situation of no home healthcare visits. Thus, no home healthcare visits were both necessary and sufficient conditions for serious falls. The second equation represents cases where no home healthcare visits and poor coordination and balance combined in cases of serious falls (both conditions are necessary but not sufficient conditions for serious falls). In the third equation, either of two causes—no healthcare home visits or poor coordination and balance—were linked to serious falls (both conditions are sufficient but not necessary). In the fourth equation, there are two different combinations linked to serious falls: serious falls occurred in cases of no

Example: Logical equations, necessary and sufficient conditions, and policy-making *(continued)*

home visits for those with poor coordination and balance, and they also occurred in cases where the patient was widowed and living alone and wore high heels. The fourth equation shows that none of the four conditions are either necessary or sufficient causes of the outcome: it suggests complex causality.[161] Thus, none of the conditions acted as causes in all instances of serious falls, nor does the data suggest that any of these conditions acted on its own to produce serious falls.

The first equation suggests a simple policy action: more funding for home healthcare visits, especially for those at risk of serious falls. The fourth equation suggest that policy responses will need to engage with a more complex causality because there is not a single homogenous cause or set of causes acting independently. It suggests that policy responses will need to be designed to ensure that interventions bring together different kinds of teams of health and allied social services practitioners to respond to the configurational causality at work in conditions present in serious falls.

Stage three: challenging the results

The third stage of a QQA-based falls prevention study would be evaluation of the results of these tests, in ways that challenge any tendencies to simplification of complex causality. This would involve testing the understandings about the causes of falls that seem suggested by the study, in the light of the larger body of evidence from the falls prevention literature. One possible technique might be to conduct an adjunct QQA analysis of falls data from a falls clinic in another (metropolitan) region, using a truth table and including summaries of falls cases. Such adjunct tests could be designed to test findings in the original study about what conditions are necessary and sufficient (or neither) for serious falls. The 'set-theoretic' statements from the two datasets could then be compared with those from the original dataset to see if the conclusions drawn from the primary study really are supportable, and what this means for policy-making and practice.

In summary, this third stage of a QQA-based falls prevention study would be testing the findings by seeking out opportunities for their falsification, leading to new findings, discarding of some findings, nuancing of others, and so on.

This third stage would provide an opportunity to build the currency and legitimacy of the study for community falls prevention policy and practice.

Research transfer into policy and practice does not always offer opportunities for practitioners and community stakeholders to be part of the testing of findings. Yet before they can act on them in high stakes contexts, community stakeholders need to have confidence in the accuracy of findings for their own contexts. QQA offers some scope for building this confidence in the contextual authenticity of findings through processes of seeking falsification.

Stage four: translating QQA findings into policy

A critical challenge would remain for the team once the research endeavour is over: to translate the research findings into policy and practice. That task involves choosing a falls intervention that is particularly well suited to meet the needs of that rural community. In practice, this will involve combining different elements of different interventions to tailor-make a holistic programme and multi-service strategy for that community, consistent with best practice in responding to falls prevention. How can the QQA research information obtained by the community-research team be used to make such decisions? The set-theoretic statements provided by the QQA study will suggest which conditions have been working in that rural community as necessary or sufficient conditions (or neither) for different types of falls linked to different conditions. However, the body of information about falls interventions exists in diverse forms that present particular problems for matching these interventions to what a community knows about the needs of its clients—in this case what the QQA study is suggesting.

One solution for the researcher is to do a meta-analysis of the information about the falls interventions using the QQA method. That is, the researcher could work with practitioners to construct a 'truth table' classifying each intervention recorded in the research literature as a case in terms of falls-relevant factors studied and its (claimed and validated) outcomes for clients. One additional attribute of interest will be the degree of evidence supporting the intervention: criteria for deciding this can be developed as part of the rules for classification for the 'truth table'. If the interventions recorded in the literature are sufficiently diverse, the cases (interventions) can be rationalized into logical equations or set-theoretic relationships. The community research team can then look for good matches between the set-theoretic statements produced by their study (i.e. conditions linking serious falls to particular risk factors in that community of clients) and the set-theoretic statements about the interventions considered as cases (.i.e. with attributes or conditions associated with particular outcomes). Policy decisions about which interventions to fund in that community could be made accordingly.

Other possible applications of QQA

The hypothetical just explored made no claims for the generalizability of findings from a QQA study. Rather, it suggested that such a study might help summarize contextual factors in ways that can lead to a better match between a particular community's needs and health interventions that have been validated in properly conducted randomized studies. However, the value of Charles Ragin's work does not lie only in micro-policy for community health interventions. Lesson-drawing using small numbers of cases is often a critical challenge for other levels and kinds of policy development.[206] There are many other possible applications of Ragin's trans-disciplinary approach to health policy, such as:

- in reviewing features of best practice health services in different systems i.e. comparative analyses of different health models considered as configurational cases

- in examining a single sensational hospital error case in a region, and comparing it to other such unusual cases in other systems, with a view to local system reform

- as an adjunct to randomized clinical studies conducted for policy, to test and refine hypotheses, including as part of the studying sub-groups or unusual cases normally not well-treated in classical experimental designs

- in researching media accounts of problems experienced by a local hospital, with a view to developing internal organizational policy on media relations.

Such small-N methods can also be helpful in pilot studies of new innovations, before major investments are made, so that policy-makers can better learn about what might be possible.[206] In fact, the possible applications are limited only by the researcher's imagination and the needs of the policy situation. The fact that Ragin's methods are not well-known to health policy-makers will present barriers for communicating their results. So also will the idea that there may be an alternative to the usual statistical methods and 'trust in numbers'. Readers will also want to consult critiques of the method that suggest it needs to be developed in ways that focus on how to prioritize the many necessary but not sufficient conditions such studies may produce.[206] This hypothetical has also suggested that great care must be taken to ensure the research findings from QQA studies are fit for purpose. A QQA study in one context does not make for universal truths that can be applied to another. However, the method may be well worth the investment in learning and explaining it, especially for small-N policy contexts where traditional qualitative and quantitative methods cannot engage with the need for both rich and systematically developed under-standings of possible underlying causal mechanisms.

Recommended reading

Ragin C. Fuzzy-Set Social Science. Chicago, The University of Chicago Press, 2000.

Readers should also consult references listed on Charles Ragin's website at http://www.u.arizona.edu/~cragin/cragin/ as well as the linked website for methodologies for cross-case analysis and small-N studies: http://www.compasss.org.

Chapter 6

Consensus-building for health policy

Overview

This chapter highlights different approaches for conducting powerful community consultations for evidence-based health policy. It explores the strengths and weaknesses of different approaches to consensus-building, which includes delivering valid data about community opinion on different policy options (consensus-finding), as well as helping develop community consensus about a particular policy option (consensus-making). The chapter offers discussion of the blend of technical research and people skills needed in conducting such consultations, as well as the ethical dimensions of such research.

The importance of participative research for health policy

... some of our more interesting public policy innovations have been through looking at an issue with a slightly different lens, or coming at it from a completely different angle using the research . . . it could also be triggered by a more anecdotal approach . . . talking to different people or consulting stakeholders who offered perspectives from different industries or different areas of policy work. And then to stress test that in order to see what are its strengths and weaknesses, before scaling it up into a national policy . . .

(health agency CEO)

Effective implementation of policy-relevant research is about bringing together rigorous methods for data collection and analysis with strategic approaches to building valid and credible evidence for policy decision-making. Health policy has specific histories of community engagement and particular stakeholder cultures. These bring distinctive challenges to the tasks of consensus-building through community consultations.

In many countries, policy directives place an impost on researchers to ensure community and patient involvement in the development of healthcare services and policy.[207] For example, in the United Kingdom, and following on from the exhortations of the White Paper *Modernising Government*,[208] the Cabinet Office report *Professional Policy Making for the Twenty First Century* described good evidence-based policy-making as taking an inclusive approach to community stakeholders, especially minorities.[44] However, a recent study of consumer involvement in NHS research found only 17% of NHS researchers were actively involving consumers, despite strong government policies advocating this involvement.[209]

There are many reasons to include strong consensus-finding and consensus-making elements in research for health policy-makers. In policy such community numbers 'talk' often much more eloquently than the results of the most elegant structural equation modelling. Participatory research approaches are important for building the relevance, political acceptability, and usefulness of research generally, not just research for health policy.[106] An exclusive reliance on scientific research approaches such as cost effectiveness, or operations research, or risk modelling would not provide the insight into community values and interests that is obtained from community-based research.[210]

Thus, community-based research has strategic value. The chapter on deciphering the policy problem referred to how the policy problem is defined by opposing interest groups. There will be different accounts of the cause and nature of the policy problem and its solutions held by different individuals and groups. Research for health policy is often about deciphering what are the opposing definitions of the policy problem and how they may be reconciled through a process of information sharing, negotiation, and solutions finding with these different interests.

The actors within institutions are also known to play a powerful role in shaping policy. They may use explicit and implicit organizational rules and conventions to shape the nature of the policy problem and solutions and how it is understood.[211] Thus, an effective notion of consensus-building should include the idea of the community of actors within the organization inhabited by policy decision-makers:

> I met a couple of captains of industry and I said, 'When you do mergers and takeovers explain to me your processes and the work that you do.' And they explained in detail the steps they went through and the amount of research they did, and then the positioning of their team when they met the other team. So that it was clearly understood by their corporate team: when they sat and planned the future of their company it was clearly articulated; it could be clearly articulated by any of that team member in negotiations of takeovers or in expansion of a joint arrangement.
>
> Policy-makers don't do that. We tend to develop a view based on a piece of work that comes to us in any form, and then we make some personal judgements around what we believe are the points for which we can deliver, and the points for which we could

realign resources or argue for additional resources. And that becomes the basis of the way that we then start to develop a framework for reform. But it's not consistent across the whole organisation, it is consistent out of the executive unit and then it becomes mandated through the organisation . . . But the work has not been done across the layers, nor has it involved all of the critical stakeholders from frontline deliverers to the data collection people through to the finance people through to the HR people . . . What are the considerations I need to give to our data people because if we want to have an evidence-based approach to this do we have the systems that will support that approach? And in terms of the frontline workers, what are the challenges in engaging and bringing into this the frontline workers who have to do the implementation of the initiative? Once the administration is layered across, then the challenging part is the community.

(health agency CEO)

It is sometimes claimed that the highly technical nature of health data and issues, such as bioethics, means that effective community consultation is unachievable. It is true that sometimes being more knowledge about issues such as bioethics can make people more distrustful.[212] However, even here, policymaking agencies have demonstrated great interest in at least the appearance of public consultation.[212] In practice, the most technical area of health involves values of some kind or another and it is in this space (at least) that community consultation can be developed. The following quotation offers an example of how scholars in the discipline of geography have described the importance of a certain style of participative research for making democracy meaningful:

> Over the last decade, policymakers and politicians have been forced to acknowledge that the institutions of representative democracy no longer secure the unquestioning support of civil society. Command and control strategies of policymaking have become a high risk strategy for governments, especially when dealing with complex and fiercely contested scientific-technological innovations such as nuclear energy and genetically modified organisms, and the need to shift to more sustainable patterns of consumption and production. We have been playing a role, alongside colleagues in geography . . . and in other academic disciplines . . . in making the case for more deliberative and inclusive democratic practices for two reasons: first to 'open up' problem framings to a wider range of perspectives and experiences; second to achieve more robust decisions through incorporation of values and knowledges beyond those of the normal science-policy community.[213](p. 276)

Key ideas

Many public policies have failed because they did not adequately reflect community norms and values. Researchers and policy-makers do not necessarily understand the issues at stake, the perceptions, values and often hidden agendas of individuals and stakeholders in the wider community.[214]

Policy-makers may be elected representatives but that does not mean that they can make sound decisions without access to systematic information about community views and opinions that can be used to 'democratize' the policy-making process.[210]

In short, policy-making can be far more powerful when it accounts for all the players on the policy-stage: the policy actors within the organization where the decision may be made, as well as the wider community of opinion.

The role of the community in consultations

We have a technique here we call the 'virtual community advisory committee' where we engage the community in a variety of ways. These are people who may have approached us either by writing to us a letter of complaint or a letter of appreciation, or by simply responding to advertisements that we have around about the opportunity to join in a virtual advisory group. We can have about seven or eight hundred people on file, who have had experience with a hospital or a product, who we will engage in these kinds of discussions. This is the way that we approach issues. So if we're looking at changing a service delivery model or if we're looking at other changes in what we're offering we'll run this by these sorts of groups first.

(health agency CEO)

The community can be conceptualized as including those who form the 'body politic': the group of stakeholders who have political value for the policy decision-maker. This may include everyone from experts or knowledge brokers who have specialized knowledge, to lay people with very limited knowledge of the policy issues.

The community-based literature also includes consideration of ways of conceptualizing the role of the community in consultations. Community participation is advocated by very different political interests and can be imbued with those different ideologies, from those of the far right to those of the far left.[215] This will shape how the research is designed and implemented. For example, the community can be positioned as having a decision-making or information-exchanging role in the policy process, as citizens, or they can be positioned as being part of a needs assessment or community development exercise.[126] In policy contexts where such 'numbers count', community members frequently need to be treated as citizens with a strategic information-giving role, such that the researcher is acting as a conduit.

Effective consultation also involves differentiating between different groups: users with direct experience of a policy at implementation level, citizens with a broader view, minority groups who may experience problems of access to health services, stakeholder groups such as representative organizations, pressure groups, and ad hoc groups, as well as internal organizational staff at all levels.[216]

The policy literature is characterized by three kinds of ideas about the involvement of the community in research for policy:

1 As an empowerment of local communities to take command of a policy agenda.
2 As a practice of co-opting community members into an existing agenda.
3 As a cynical public relations exercise justifying a predetermined policy decision.[215]

This kind of theorizing of community involvement characterizes Arnstein's much-discussed 'ladder' of community involvement which suggests that the greater the level of community ownership of the research process, the better.[217] However, in practice, all parties to the consultations hold some kind of power and the context will vary the nature of this power and effective styles of community participation. Accordingly, the literature suggests that it may not be right to idealize community participation in terms of levels of participation, as if the greater the participation, the higher the quality of involvement.[209]

Key ideas

For policy-making contexts Arnstein's ladder has the disadvantage that it brings implications of moral virtue to degrees of community ownership of decision-making, as if community participation was an end in itself. Policy decision-makers may see no virtue in a high level of community participation or a process of 'empowerment' that results in a decision that is ultimately unworkable, including for the community itself.

This does not mean that *a priori* notions of process are unimportant: it is certainly critical to both actually consult and be seen to consult. It does mean that process is not the only goal in policy-relevant research. What also matters is the success for the community of the policy option produced by such consultative processes.

The devotion in this book of a separate chapter to community consensus-building does not mean that community consultation will or should fit neatly into a discrete stage of research for policy. Community members can be involved at all stages of the research from conceptualization of the policy problem, review of the literature, research design and data collection to dissemination of the research. This chapter focuses more on the value of a systematic primary data collection phase that allows the gathering of information about solutions to policy problems from diverse stakeholders. It is sometimes but not always useful to conduct this data collection after the literature review is largely completed.

Critical aspects of community consensus-building

'Consensus-building' is a term that includes 'consensus-finding' and 'consensus-making'. Unless areas of consensus are found or identified, the researcher cannot work to consensus-make. In this book both processes are represented as ideally occurring from the early stages of diagnosing the research to the latter stages of disseminating the research. However, the formal collection of primary data collection from the community can be conceptualized as a critical event in consensus-building.

'Consensus-finding' is diagnostic. It is about finding out what the community already knows and thinks about policy options i.e. existing community attitudes and definitions of the policy problem. However, it is not enough to ask the community what it thinks. The policy-relevant researcher must actively facilitate the community's opinion-making through consultative research practices that draw heavily on negotiation and conflict resolution skills. 'Consensus-making' positions the researcher as an active agent for change, using research processes to develop community views around a particular policy problem and its solutions. Consensus-making is a critical skill in policy-relevant research, which is often adversarial, even (and sometimes especially) when commissioned by policy decision-makers.

Consensus-finding may be diagnostic but it should not be conceptualized as the simpler task. Unreflective and methodologically unsophisticated surveying of public opinion may lead to high stakes errors in how community views are represented. The same individuals, groups, and communities can hold contradictory attitudes. The views can be pragmatic, economic, ideological, political, prejudiced, evangelical, historical, cultural, 'ignorant', and so on. Consensus-finding involves not simply describing community views but also providing explanations of why those views are held. Where there are differences in views, the dynamics of the differences need to be understood.[218]

Consensus-making is not about identifying recalcitrant members of the public who should be 'educated' to take other views as part of some deficit model.[218] Consensus-making involves using understandings of disputes and differences to facilitate and shape enlightened community consensus about the policy problem and its solutions. It draws heavily upon conflict resolution skills.

Key ideas

Critical tasks in community consensus-building (consensus-finding and consensus-making) over the term of the policy-relevant research are:

♦ identifying stakeholders

> **Key ideas** *(continued)*
>
> ◆ using groups and individuals to help diagnose the policy problem and its causes
>
> ◆ enlarging stakeholder understandings of the policy problem
>
> ◆ developing and negotiating the policy solutions with stakeholders
>
> ◆ obtaining stakeholder feedback on the report and further developing it in the light of that feedback.[214]

The formal data collection phase involving the community tends to make its greatest contribution by way of using community members to diagnose and develop shared understandings of the policy problem, as well as develop and negotiate the possible policy options with stakeholders.

Policy networks: a key challenge of community consensus-building

As has been noted, the policy literature emphasizes the importance of policy networks which operate in direct and indirect, as well as unintentional, ways to shape policy.[214] Government, especially in democratic systems, may be the primary actor in public health policy but is not a 'black box that directs policy-making in a unilateral and temporally linear way'[214] (p. 189). Government operates in a web of relationships or networks. Part of the challenge of interacting with organizations and individuals in such policy-making networks is that they may have political or other responsibilities for, or degrees of ownership of, the policy problem. They may also be variously implicated in the cause of the problem.[214, 219] Each will also have their own political agendas. The existence of policy networks suggests that community opinion is not a malleable entity. Accordingly, it is important not to overstate or understate the capacity of research to build consensus. Chapter 3 offers ideas for identifying and mapping policy networks.

The methods discussed later in this chapter build on that discussion to offer tools for identifying and engaging with these networks in ways that can help maximize consensus.

The ethical researcher for health policy: a working definition

There are different specialized areas of ethics literature on public policy-making, including in health. However, ethics for health policy analysis is not well-represented in the literature.[220] How should researchers behave in community consultations when faced with the particular ethical dilemmas of health policy-making? Most researchers these days operate within ethical frameworks for the general conduct of research. However, there is no explicit international ethical framework adapted for community-based research for health policy. Notwithstanding, a number of ethical responsibilities can be identified, the most important of which may be accurately conveying community views, whether they emerge from consensus-making or consensus-building where the researcher has been a more active agent.

The ethical researcher for health policy does not necessarily need to believe that the public health policy options under investigation are the best ones for a community. One reason for this in public sector research is that the researcher's ideas of 'the common good' may not be compatible with the model of impartial service idealized in traditional Westminster concepts of the public service. In this framework, what matters is the impartiality of the service rendered to government, and through government, to the community. The public sector researcher is thus not an academic invested with disciplinary expertise that allows him or her to arbitrate on what is for the common good. In a simplistically idealized democratic system, the policy-maker is the nominee of a government democratically elected to make decisions about the common good. If, in a democratic system, few believe senior policy-makers are fully committed to the common good that does not mean researchers can easily determine it, even if they are disciplinary experts.

In practice, most policy options being considered belong in a grey zone, and it is the function of the researcher to find out in what ways they might meet different kinds of public goods.

Key ideas

In this book, the ethical role of researchers is represented as being about facilitating democratic policy-making through rigorous, accountable and valid research practices. Taking this principle as the guiding beacon, many other ethical responsibilities become evident.

For example, wherever possible, community participants should also receive feedback about the outcomes of the research exercise. This is critical not simply for the standard ethical reasons. Researchers for policy may want to build their social capital in communities of interest by ensuring that they gain a reputation for delivering research that does not disappear into a 'black hole'. This means they should communicate their results, even if these results are limited to the fact that a policy report has been successfully submitted rather than the fact that it resulted in specific successful changes to policy.

Using the principle of facilitating democratic policy-making as a guide, it can also be seen that community-based research for health policy-making involves a responsibility to ensure that all members of a community (such as those with disabilities who experience particular problems of access) have equal opportunity to participate in the consultations.

Inclusiveness in community consultations: equity and quality

... if you're trying to reach a group then you need to go where they are and you need to focus the discussions in a way that's appropriate for that group of people

(health agency CEO)

The observation 'Don't forget the margins' is right because if you take the approach that this is just about getting a piece of policy through the door, well you do that on majorities and just get it done. If this is actually about designing your health care system to meet the needs of people whoever and wherever they are, you have got to design policy for everybody, which is then about how you develop independent pieces of packages of care for individual clients. And so you have to go to the single voice.

(health agency CEO)

As the earlier discussion suggested, quality policy options for particular communities developed without meeting the challenges of including their experiences, values, and opinions are unlikely to work. The researcher for policy also has an ethical duty to ensure that disability, gender, age, economic status, race, ethnicity, and other characteristics of individuals and groups do not become barriers to their participation in policy-making. Different strategies will need to be employed to ensure the high quality valid participation of people experiencing particular kinds of disadvantage.

Key ideas

Equity in community consultations is not about using the same approach to include everyone. It may involve using different approaches for different individuals and groups, to ensure that everyone has equal opportunity to participate. In a sentence, the literature suggests that viewing each community group as unique and tailor-making research approaches with a strong, well-informed sense of 'other' is an important prerequisite for achieving inclusive research for policy.

Achieving this ideal of equal opportunity to participate presents particular ethical and research design challenges. There is a great deal of research that suggests that particular groups, such as aboriginal peoples, have experienced considerable oppression through research practices that position them as objects of study, rather than as 'experts of their lives' who are able to help others understand the historical, social and economic conditions relevant to their lived experience.[221] For community members experiencing disadvantage, the ethical issues will be about how their data will be used to shape policy that may directly affect them in ways that research for academic publication would not and in ways the researcher is unlikely to be able to control. Researchers will need to develop and adapt consultation styles that account for such issues, and actively facilitate the participation of these groups and the validity and quality of their input.

In meeting such challenges, researchers for policy may want to review the relevant guidelines for consulting with specific groups, including disadvantaged groups. For example, in Australia there are very specific guidelines for the conduct of research involving indigenous people published by the National Health and Medical Council. These offer a gold standard for those working with such groups. The research literature also contains some helpful models for research practice in this area.[222] For example, a useful model for working with people with learning disabilities and severe mental health problems has been developed using simplified line drawings and pictures that can be used in interviews with clients in these groups.[207]

Such guidelines and literature also include suggestions to work directly with representatives of disadvantaged groups. The value of this cannot be overstated. Many researchers for policy nowadays will work with a task group that is designed to include representatives of disadvantaged groups. These representatives can help ensure approaches and instruments adapted from the international literature are in fact valid for the local groups and their contexts.

Key practical strategy

The advice of community leaders can help ensure researchers are familiar with community protocols for working with particular disadvantaged groups and data collection tools are culturally appropriate. Community elders can also help ensure there are iterative approaches to the development of findings, through successive group and/or individual meetings designed to create a sense of ownership of the data collected from these groups. Particular measures such as honoraria may be appropriate to ensure that the experience of research in that community is of

> **Key practical strategy** *(continued)*
>
> 'giving something back.' Feedback loops to the community need to be given careful consideration; they are especially critical for groups that have historical experiences of being ignored and marginalized, such as aboriginal peoples.[221]

The literature also offers the advice that researchers involving such groups in consultations will need to allow for the resource intensive nature of the process.[207] However, the investment is well worth it. Many policy-makers want and need research that conveys the views and experiences of all community groups. They are aware that while equity and quality in policy-relevant research may not be exactly the same things, they are related.

Further discussion of practices for ensuring diversity in community-based methods for health research is given in the monograph *Community-Based Participatory Research for Health*.[223]

Guiding principles for designing community consultations

There is no single model or method of community engagement that represents best practice, since what works will depend on the context. However, the OECD as well as governments in some countries have produced practical and in-principle introductory guides for community consultation for public policy-making, designed specifically for policy-makers and those who deliver research to them.[216, 224] These can offer a basis for designing quality consultations. There is also some consensus in the scholarly literature about the principles that ought to guide the design of consumer research. Collectively these suggest that

- the roles of participants, researchers, and policy-makers need to be agreed upon, and the objectives and limitations of consultation should be declared in advance
- participation must be planned so that adequate financial, human, and technical support is available to support the consultation process
- the different knowledge and skills of the participants should be valued
- participants should have the training and support they need to properly participate
- participants should be involved as early as possible in the development of policy solutions

- researchers should ensure they have the necessary skills to involve participants
- participants should be involved in decisions about who should be consulted and should be kept informed of the research progress
- participant involvement should be appropriately documented in the research reports: it should be objectively portrayed and be complete
- the research findings should be available to participants in accessible formats that allow for open external scrutiny of the use of community views.[209, 216, 224]

A more detailed discussion of principles for, and ways of framing, community consultations is offered by the monograph *Community Based Participatory Research for Health*.[223]

Pitfalls of community consultation

Researchers should also be aware of the ways in which community consultations can create problems for policy-makers. In the UK, the Cabinet Office report *Professional Policy Making for the Twenty First Century* describes the pitfalls of consultation for policy-makers as including

- delay and administrative overload
- creating a focus for certain community interests to mobilize resistance against efforts to progress an issue and produce unrepresentative views if particular stakeholders manage to dominate the consultation process
- raising impossible expectations that all views will be acted upon.[44]

The strategies in this chapter aim to help the researcher develop a plan for the consultations which is time effective and inclusive of all views. The section on community distrust later in this chapter explores how to manage expectations about what the research can and should do for community members wishing to be heard by policy-makers.

However, some of the reasons that community consultations are unproductive or even a liability for policy-makers relates to the basic quality of the research methods used. For example, if the methods of data collection include a survey that is not based on an understanding of how question wording and order can affect how respondents answer the survey form, or an understanding of basic sampling methods, the data are likely to be unusable. If interviews are not done with an awareness of best practices in interviewing techniques, including standardization of questions, the interview data may also be seriously flawed. The data may also be compromised if the consultation method is not designed to fit the purpose, which will vary depending on the stage of the policy-making cycle involved: the community may be involved in identifying or analysing the nature of the policy problem, developing the policy options, as well as implementing and monitoring the policy.[216] Consultation using electronic technologies ('e-consultation') can also do more harm than good if protocols are not developed and moderators are not used appropriately. Resources developed by the Cabinet Office of the Blair government as part of its efforts to develop evidence-based policy offer an introduction to such basic matters of quality and validity in community-based data collection and research methods, as well as links to other resources[82, 216]—topics which this book is not designed to treat. Community consultations for policy-makers are best designed and led by researchers who have knowledge and experience in basic research methods, and ideally in the more advanced methods for consultation detailed in this chapter.

Action research frameworks and tools for designing community consultations

There are specific action-based frameworks and tools available for community based research. Some of these are highlighted in subsequent text here. The emphasis is on broad approaches with applications across different sub-disciplines of health. However, researchers should be aware that in some areas, such as bioethics, special tools have been developed to measure community attitudes.[212] These can be invaluable, even if only used as a point of departure for research designs. As noted previously, there are also introductory toolkits for community consultation for public policy-making produced by different organizations and governments such as the UK Cabinet Office resources and the OECD.[216, 224] The UK government has also published papers on public involvement in health that include lists of resources such as government policy and guidelines on community participation as well as the websites of organizations concerned with public involvement.[225] Researchers might also like to consult a useful information toolkit on techniques for conducting community consultations developed by Health Canada.[226] Such toolkits also suggest how in different countries public consultations operate within particular policy frameworks for participative government that shape the methods of consultation that should be used.

Action research approaches offer one way of designing community consultations for health policy-making. However, they are not necessarily specifically designed to meet the needs of research for policy-making and there are many areas of health policy where such approaches have not yet been applied.[227]

Community-Based Participatory Research (CBPR) is one kind of action research approach that has been used in developing public health policy. It is a collaborative approach for achieving community-based change aimed at community health and health disparities, typically around a single micro-policy challenge.[228] The approach is defined more by its orientation to community participation in problem-solving using both qualitative and quantitative methods than by a specific distinctive method. The research methods are designed to be educative and act as agents of change by involving community members in the research and giving them ownership of the research process. It is thought that people who reflect on health information about best practice and are involved in research on their own community health issues may be more likely to be motivated to change their own health behaviours and that of the groups to which they belong. In such a research approach the process of research is itself the action for achieving the outcome.[228]

The PANDA (Participatory Appraisal of Needs and Development of Action) approach is similar to other action research approaches in the sense that it is not a method as such but rather a framework under which many different research techniques can be grouped. It emphasizes the creative combining of different methods to build community relationships and collect views on community conditions, such as problem-structuring approaches and participatory appraisal methods (mapping, diagramming, and matrix scoring, to understand people's needs, their organizations, and their past experiences).[126, 215, 229] The emphasis is on iterative 'bottom-up' participatory planning and solutions development. Options are formulated, evaluated and selected. This approach has potential for helping develop evidence-based understandings of community needs, especially for politically sensitive policy-making. The main value of the PANDA approach for research for health policy is that it offers suggestions for

- diverse research techniques for consensus-building (such as the use of visual tools for maximizing participation)
- different combinations of research techniques designed to meet the needs of different groups and
- different kinds of roles that can be adopted by the researcher as facilitator.[229]

The PANDA approach can be particularly helpful where the policy options under consideration require the community to own, internalize, and act upon or implement the options. Readers might like to consult the manual produced by White, Taket, and Gibbons for further details: it has been used in developing countries, as well as the United Kingdom.[229, 230]

Participatory Action Research (PAR) is another related action research approach that can involve both decision-makers and community stakeholders in a staged reflection and dialogue that help generate knowledge for action and change. It can be used to focus on any end, such as priority setting for scarce resources, combining programme budgeting and resource priority-setting approaches.[57] It combines purposive sampling of stakeholders and thematic coding schemes of qualitative data from such data collection techniques as focus groups and interviews.[57]

Community mapping

The aforementioned description of action research approaches suggests an important aspect of community consultations: mapping the needs and resources of a community. This has evolved into a fine art form in the applied social science literature. It involves community needs assessment, as well as community capacity or asset inventories.

Key practical strategy

Community needs assessment involves mapping the perceived and actual needs of a community. Community capacity and asset inventories involve using a wide range of data gathering methods to create a list of the material and human resources of a community. This can be part of the process of establishing the sustainability of different possible policy options explored in Chapter 4.

This mapping can be done by researchers and/or community members. Ideally though, it will involve dialogue between both researchers and community members as part of consensus-building about policy problems and solutions. More innovative approaches to mapping community needs, capacities and assets can involve using the creative arts: community murals, workshops on art and literature, as well as film and dramatizations of community issues.[223] These can help create media through which diverse community groups can express their needs and capacities.

A tool for identifying stakeholders and their issues: Q-methodology

... it's very easy for policy-makers who may disagree with the findings to discredit stakeholder-based work, so I guess drawing the tent as broadly as possible would be an obvious bit of advice ... and probably touching base early on in the design with who the likely opponents or nay sayers will be and having them suggest people who need to be included in the stakeholder process might help ...

(health services CEO)

Stakeholders for data collection (not just early stage deciphering of the policy challenge) can be identified with reference to informal sources such as policy networks, media coverage of the issue, previous applied policy research, and so on, using snowball sampling in which stakeholders so identified are asked to add to the list.[214, 219]

Preliminary mapping of the policy issues attached to particular stakeholders can also be very helpful prior to the larger formal data collection exercise involving the wider community. The documents produced by stakeholders—from any available internal memos to policy discussion papers and reports—can be collected to obtain information about how community members understand the policy problem.[214] Such excavation needs to be time sensitive as documents may be out-of-date even if very recent. Media coverage can also be used to add to the preliminary map of community views on the policy problem at stake, though of course, the media can never be considered a transparent window through which community views can be observed.[214] It is important to take a historical view when excavating public opinion, by tracing the evolution of particular policy arguments and problems over time, in the language produced by different community stakeholders, including the anecdotal accounts given by contacts in policy networks. This kind of exercise will never be definitive though it may powerfully position the researcher for the tasks of community consultation—even if it simply identifies what is not known about who thinks what.

'Q-methodology' is a methodology for community consultations that has been used to identify the different kinds of values revealed by the differing language styles that different groups in a community may hold. It has been largely applied in environmental policy and politics.[218] It is based on the idea that individuals who share particular ways of using language reflecting shared values can be identified and can be differentiated from those who share other values and thus ways of using language. This is helpful for understanding which groups in a community believe what and why. Use of 'Q-methodology' involves several steps:

1 Collecting samples of language of different groups (for example, through media clippings and/or interviews and focus groups etc.).

2 Identification and sorting by the researcher of significant statements using a matrix.

3 Community members who self-identify as objectors or supporters of particular policy options are then invited to agree or disagree with the statements so identified using rules that only allow them to, for example 'most agree' or 'most disagree', and so on with a certain number of statements, thus facilitating more subtle understandings of the nature of views held by them.

4 The sorting of statements that has taken place is further progressed using the relevant software which applies statistical techniques such as factor analysis to identify participants (by groups) who sorted the statements in particular ways.

5 The researcher then interprets the statistical analysis so produced using further data such as post-sort interviews in ways that lead to identification of particular distinctive ways of using language associated with particular clusters of supporting and objecting groups.

6 After these clusters of language by supporting and objecting groups are identified, the interpretation of them by the researcher is explored in focus group meetings of objectors, supporters, and a mixed group.[218]

The resulting data analysis using this 'Q-methodology' provides a table labelling the different kinds of objectors and supporters, and the statements that had the most agreement and disagreement in these sub-groups.[218] Thus this method allows researchers to explore the many ways in which community members say 'yes' to different policy options, as well as the many ways in which they may say 'no'.[218] This information can be used to design approaches to developing community consensus around the particular policy options.

Such a method might be useful to do prior to the formal data collection exercise involving the community, by way of analysis of the status quo of such views. That is, Q-methodology can be used as a platform for designing more deliberative approaches i.e. as a device for seeking 'first stage' community views about the policy options after the researcher has had preliminary discussions with policy-makers and undertaken the literature reviews.

The strength of the Q-methodology is that it allows a more systematic approach to analysing the subtleties of community views than some narrative approaches, using both qualitative and quantitative techniques. Too many approaches to seeking community consensus do not try to first understand the anatomy of both opposing and supporting views: the subtle differences between those who may share opposing views or share supporting views. Such an approach also allows questioning of implicit assumptions of policy-makers about their communities, which may themselves be the barriers to developing better policy options.[218]

Practical techniques for maximizing community participation

Obtaining desirable levels of participation of stakeholders in research for health policy presents specific challenges. For example, involving medical professionals in participative research is known to be very challenging, and there are documented studies of what makes a difference to response rates, such as working through professional associations.[231] Typically, community engagement projects will also involve a reference group drawn from relevant stakeholder groups. This can be a valuable resource for advice about relevant techniques for maximizing community participation. This section highlights a few techniques for maximizing participative research for health policy, as well as their challenges.

Community forums and panels

> . . . one of the methods that we've found useful in terms of generating the right kind of message is engagement of community advisory committees who actually serve almost as focus groups for listening to data, listening to their peers, listening to information that we're going to be putting forward in terms of changes in the approach we're taking. Before we actually take those to the stakeholders we'll try them on our community advisory committee as an example.
>
> (health agency CEO)

Community forums can involve different formats for different purposes. An introduction to such forums is given in the toolkit for community consultations produced by the UK government's Cabinet Office *Viewfinder: A Policy-Maker's Guide to Public Involvement*.[216] Town meetings are a frequently used mechanism for bringing researchers, residents, health workers, local community leaders, and others from relevant community organizations together to achieve broad input. Such forums need careful planning to work; planning that ideally includes some consideration of the experience of others as represented in the research literature generally, as well as the experience of the local community. Particular strategies can make an enormous difference to the success of a town meeting. For example, the press can be used to publicize the event before and after, and make a critical difference to community dialogue about and awareness of the issues.[232] Other kinds of community forums can be created in the format of open conferences and workshops. Symposia can also be used to bring together research experts, funders and policy-makers, as well as other specialist stakeholders to do particular tasks such as deciding the research design for examining the effectiveness and translation of complex, multi-level health interventions.[106] Retreats with key stakeholder representatives can offer more intensive opportunities for consensus-making.

The use of panels offers another kind of format for community forums. One model of this format for achieving community participation is 'Participatory Policy Analysis' (PPA). This involves using panels of community members who have been selected randomly from a larger body of community members.

The aim is to facilitate a 'two-way' street for exchange of information: from policy-makers to community and vice versa. The panel reflects on the policy decisions, providing a supposedly impartial representation of values and views in the wider community.[210] There are other variations of community panels such as 'citizens' juries' which involve 12–20 people from the community meeting to hear expert witnesses and decide a course of action over a series of days.[82]

Many kinds of policy problems will also involve obtaining the opinions of an expert group. The 'policy Delphi method' has been adapted for these kinds of data gathering challenges.[233] This method allows information to be gathered from experts that cannot so easily be gathered from literature reviews. The policy Delphi method combines both qualitative and quantitative methods. The policy options under consideration are put before the experts; information about their value, impact, and so on are then gathered.[233] However, the aim of the exercise is not necessarily to arrive at consensus (as in the traditional version of the Delphi method), but rather to obtain more information about the pros and cons of different policy options. Questionnaires with Likert scales and open-ended items, as well as focus groups can be used. Data from one stage of data collection are used to develop the data-gathering instruments for the second stage, to facilitate stability of opinions on a policy option. The first questionnaire, however, is based on a literature review.[233]

Of course, there are many opportunities for gathering community opinion opened up by the electronic age. Electronic community forums can be created through, for example, video-conferencing using multiple-sites, or the creation of discussion lists, electronic letterboxes, on-line live chat events, interactive games and scenarios, and other formats on internet sites. Discussion lists are sometimes used in public policy research because they allow opportunities to have extended conversations on complex policy problems. Further details about using these and other e-consultation methods are given in the introductory toolkits for community consultation developed by the Cabinet Office of the UK government as well as the OECD, which also offer references to other resources.[216, 224] Useful approaches and examples of tools for using electronic media to maximize community participation are also given in the monograph *Community-Based Participatory Research for Health*.[223] Most notable of these is an approach called 'Photovoice' which involves providing community members with cameras for recording the day-to-day realities of community experience and views. This involves a 'reality TV' approach that can promote community dialogue about policy issues and solutions. It has particular strengths as an approach for helping disadvantaged groups narrate their concerns, including for community mapping exercises.[223] However, there is a general lack of specific guidance in the literature about how e-consultation methods affect the quality and validity of data gathered. For this reason researchers may want to ensure that such data-gathering methods are supplemented with others, especially to triangulate high stakes hypotheses.

Clearly, each of these public forums brings with it sets of social protocols that can shape and limit the extent to which the forum offers insight into how the community is thinking about a particular policy problem. The medium really can be the message in community consultations. For example, electronic discussion lists can work to create spaces for certain leaders of community opinion or particular groups such as young people, but they may also work to silence those who do not use such media such as older people and those on lower incomes. Town meetings may ensure the silence of those who feel unable to take a view that is controversial to their neighbours. Deciding on the best community forum is about deciding not simply who should be heard, but also who should not be silenced.

Surveys for consensus-building

> ... to get the input on our survey we've actually had our governor send out a letter telling health care providers of the importance of this project, and I think that has enhanced the return on the survey.
>
> (health agency CEO)

Surveys for community consensus-building in the health sector present specific challenges. A review of the literature suggests that researchers may be able to maximize responses to postal questionnaires for patients (at least) by including telephone reminders and keeping questionnaires short, though no evidence was found to support the idea that incentives are helpful.[234] In at least one account, blind mass mailings of long surveys from unknown researchers to health professionals were seen as unlikely to be successful, whereas more personalized approaches such as direct telephone calling appeared more effective.[231] However, a Cochrane review suggests that there is a very low quality of evidence that telephone discussions and face-to-face group meetings actually engage consumers better than mailed surveys for the purposes of setting priorities for community health goals. This review suggests that there is very little research evidence establishing the best ways of involving consumers in healthcare decisions.[235] In the face of this lack of empirical certainty, the 'fitness for purpose' test should be applied.

Large scale surveys may be fit to be used to gather data on community opinion, especially where people may prefer to offer their views outside public forums and in a manner where their anonymity is guaranteed. However, mailed surveys may not be so helpful to building the partnership culture that is important in consensus-building. In policy-making contexts, surveys can have political repercussions that are difficult to control and manage. They may also have validity problems to do with the complexity of obtaining data about values in either a qualitative or quantitative form with 'closed questions'. In contrast to methods such as focus groups, mass mailed survey questions can suppress ambiguity and reduce the visibility of complex issues.[212] However, they can be valuable for randomized scoping of the extent and nature of particular community opinions, or for targeting groups that cannot be reached in other ways.

Semi-structured, open-ended questions can be used in randomized telephone surveys to create at least some level of personal contact with community members. Randomized telephone surveys can also be useful for handling groups of non-respondents in mass mailed surveys. Short telephone surveys may be more readily accepted by many non-responding community members who were unwilling to fill out survey forms. The telephone surveys in this situation can be designed to test the main hypotheses emerging from the mass mailed survey. In this way, researchers can be more confident that the percentage of non-respondents to a larger mailed survey did not include groups who would have responded very differently.

Few studies exist about the value of survey approaches that take advantage of electronic media, such as emailed invitations to community members to participate in online surveys. These can be very cost effective, and may work well if the online survey is short and well-designed. However, they may also suffer from the poor response rates of mailed surveys.

Ideally, researchers for policy will use third parties to help them broker higher survey response rates, such as professional associations and consumer representative organizations, employing authorities, and so on.

Researchers for policy may also be interested in taking a 'geo-spatial' approach to the task of maximizing community participation. This involves examining how to maximize community participation by considering information about the places and spaces where different groups tend to congregate at particular times. An electronic map can be developed from the different sites that are frequented by the community of opinion that the researcher is trying to target, based on such data. For example, stalls at shopping centres and malls can be used to target older or younger citizens, depending on the time of day. Such stalls are best used to build community awareness of the policy issue and the wider research exercise being conducted, through the distribution of pamphlets and making the researcher accessible to community members.

The performative aspects of consultative research

Despite their relative neglect in the health policy research literature, the performative dimensions of the researcher's role in community consultations can have an important role to play in consensus-building. These can be described as the use by the researcher of his or her physical characteristics (voice, gestures, stance, etc.) to deliver a public persona that maximizes the participation of diverse community groups.

Literature on community participation scarcely acknowledges the performative aspects of the researcher's role—as if the researcher is not also a kind of actor in a play. However, some accounts of community participation frameworks, such as the previously discussed PANDA approach, place an emphasis on the performative aspects of the researcher's role in maximizing the equity and quality of community participation.[229] In the PANDA framework for a pragmatic eclecticism in research methods, the researcher interacts with different community groups and so must take on different kinds of roles depending on the needs of those community groups. For example, the researcher may act out the role of a naïve enquirer to help open up assumptions and subjects that may not have been previously debated, or may be a provoker challenging community members to disagree.

The importance of the researcher being able to adopt these different roles and adapt his or her public persona to meet the communication needs of community groups in consultative research is described by the authors of the PANDA approach in this way:

> Different roles were used by the facilitator to encourage participants to subject any assumptions about sources of legitimation to critical evaluation, through considering aspects of the relevance, applicability, feasibility, and acceptability of the *content* under discussion to the local situation, rather than imputing these from any perception about the *standing* of the speaker.[229] (p. 161)

This suggests that varying the roles or persona the researcher adopts in interacting with community groups may be important for maximizing the validity of data obtained from community members. Another way of putting this is to say that without some consciousness of these personas, researchers may not be aware of the extent to which the data they collected from community consultations are an artefact of the person their audience supposed they were.

Taket and White also point to the importance of performative aspects of the researcher's role for maximizing the participation of different equity target groups. One example is the ways in which different physical cues and behaviours can be required to maximize communication with men and women in different cultural contexts.[229] This is something that was suggested by the earlier section on issues in including disadvantaged groups in health policy consultations.

Accordingly, rather than being beneath the attention of serious researchers, the performative aspects of the researcher's role can be considered as an important part of the work of achieving equity (inclusiveness) and quality (validity and accuracy) in consensus-finding. They can also be considered an important part of the work of brokering agreement on policy options between different groups. The confidence and trust of an audience can be gained by correctly reading its communicative style (formal to informal) and mirroring this back to that audience. Or it may be gained by recognizing that what the group wants and needs is not this mirroring but perhaps more of a leadership style of interaction in which the researcher helps the group achieve consensus by being more assertive in presenting options.

Key practical strategy

Experienced researchers for policy may respond to high conflict in community consultations by tailor-making responsive personas that help them maximize resolution and instil confidence and trust. They may spend time before the community forum event begins carefully scrutinizing the list of attendees, their backgrounds, likely relevant experiences and opinions. They may also design a format for conducting the community consultations that works to complement the performance they need to deliver.

For example, in a sensitive situation where a community is angry about a recent policy decision about their health services, the researcher may want to adopt the role of negotiator using visual representations of the content of various policy arguments along the lines of the PANDA approach. Such visual representations have been used to 'manage latent conflict and to open up a space for collaboration' by helping those involved in a conflict 'obtain some distance from the dispute' [229](p. 165).

Data collection and analysis issues for community forums

Researchers have to accept the fact that many people who are interacting with you would have a specific point of view. And they have a direction that they're trying to steer the system, that's part of the reason why they're engaged in the process. So I think it is important to understand the bias of the groups that you're interacting with.

(health agency CEO)

The mutually compatible design of qualitative and quantitative instruments for community consultations is part of the art of participative research for policy. The instruments can be designed to test key hypotheses about the nature and extent of community opinion on particular possible policy options. Quantitative instruments can be designed to supplement and triangulate findings from qualitative instruments.

Key practical strategy

The data collection can also have a heuristic function: to help community members understand and debate key policy options by inviting them into the process of consideration of the policy goals and healthcare system complexities that policy-makers may be facing.

Attention should also be paid to the graphical and typographical possibilities of these research instruments for different groups, and their potential as highly visual and interactive media. Bearing in mind the emphasis on inclusiveness previously discussed, ideas from approaches such as the PANDA framework can be used to design instruments with diagrams that facilitate the participation of diverse community members, some of whom may have literacy difficulties.[229]

There are also many practical considerations. In community forums, the researcher will want to know whether the views being collected are those of individuals or their organizations: this distinction may need to be made in the data collection techniques.[214] Even if this information is obtained, the views collected may need to be audited against documents from the stakeholder organizations so represented.[214] In large community meetings, note-taking as well as taping of responses may be necessary. The note-taker can ask speakers in both focus groups and large community meetings to identify themselves wherever necessary. This enables the paraphrased notes to be cross-checked using the taped responses.

Policy researchers advocate a form of coding for analysis of the qualitative results of community consultations, using categories established by the development of the definition of the policy problem, and available software for such qualitative analyses.[214] The interpretations of the data using these categories ought to be shared with community stakeholders to audit the researcher's readings of both qualitative and quantitative data.[214] Ideally, a number of researchers and representatives from different stakeholder groups would be used for these cross-checks to ensure readings are robust and have credibility in the wider community.

Many of the qualitative and quali-quantitative research approaches described in Chapters 4 and 5 are useful for analysis of data about community views. General guidance on analysing community views is also available in such toolkits as the Blair government's *Viewfinder: A Policy Maker's Guide to Public Involvement*.[216]

Building trust in community consultations: the roots of cynicism

> Consultation is a dreadful name for doing something to get a mandate to do something you've probably decided anyway. We often have this dilemma, and we talk about it often, about don't consult if you've made the decision or if you haven't got the ability to influence.
>
> (health agency CEO)

The focus of the discussion to this point has largely been on research techniques as well as skills of social brokering and role-playing important to community consensus-building. This suggests that consensus-building for health policy is a challenge that draws heavily on the researcher's creative design as well as people skills.

Key ideas

The challenge of cynicism in communities suggests why people skills cannot be neglected in participative research. The literature offers indications that what matters to community members is not what forum or methodology is used for participative research processes, but rather what information is shared and how it is shared among participants and decision-makers.[236]

Information-giving is critical because it allows community members to participate in reflecting on the technical complexity of issues and the creative work of policy-making.[236] However, whatever the research technique used, or its content, it must be structured in a way that allows the community to freely and frankly raise their concerns.[212] This 'openness' is critical to consensus-building, particularly given the likelihood that community members will be highly critical and discerning participants of any attempts to involve them in research. In the United Kingdom, the Cabinet Office report *Professional Policy Making for the 21st Century* described how a review of policy-making approaches in the United Kingdom suggested that consultation had in some cases been used as a means of 'flushing out' challenges to prospective policies.[44]

This kind of use of community consultation has a heavy legacy for subsequent efforts to do research with these communities. Citizen participants may also have been subjected to processes of community consultation that are simply about creating the illusion that consultation has happened. They may express their wariness of research in a certain style of apathy, either through low participation rates in the consultations or low energy levels at the research forums. As one citizen participant commented in a study of this issue 'we are becoming an apathetic society, but I think a lot of it has to do with the way we were treated last time'.[236]

The task of identifying stakeholder groups and researching their history of engagement with the policy problem, referred to earlier, is very important. Specifically, the researcher may want to find out about the history of previous attempts to consult the particular communities that are being targeted for the present consultation. Questions to ask include 'What kind of profile does this particular set of policy-makers have in this community?' There should be no assumption that cynicism is the same in every community. Research suggests that each community may have its own particular 'roots of cynicism' just as they also have their own distinctive positive experiences with policy-making consultations that can be drawn upon.[236] Positive experiences held by particular stakeholders can be a place to begin consideration of which leaders in a community can be used as 'consensus brokers'. In the light of this historical information about the experiences in the community that need careful negotiation (or adroit capitalization), further attention can be paid to getting the content and balance of information right in order to build trust and credibility.[236] This will also involve the kind of performative dimensions of research discussed previously. Researchers who hold public meetings and other participative forums will need to be skilled communicators: skilled at managing conflict, crowd control, listening, rephrasing and repeating back statements, and so on.

Key practical strategy

Inviting community members to reflect on the 'rocks and hard places' or trade-offs between different pressures and constraints that policy-makers face which can limit their ability to respond to community wishes can be a very powerful approach to building trust in that community. Such an invitation can work to position community members to make the biggest possible difference because their views include mediating factors. In this kind

Key practical strategy *(continued)*

of model of community consultation, community members are given the role of problem-solvers synthesising a range of considerations, not just information-giving about their own experiences. However, this needs to be carefully done to ensure it is successful, given the complex range of information that will need to be considered. One strategy is to invite groups of different stakeholder representatives to consider portfolios of information and provide feedback about their preferences for particular kinds of trade-offs.

The participation process should give citizens a clear purpose and have built-in accountability mechanisms that are clearly conveyed to the participants.[236] That is, participants should know not only what information is being requested but why and how that information will be used. Further to the emphasis elsewhere on feedback to research participants, it should be noted that this feedback has an important role in building trust and overcoming cynicism. This means there should be a specific process for feedback declared in advance, not simply the usual general ethical statement that recognizes participants' common right to know the results of the research project.

In declaring the purpose of the research, the researcher need not imply or support in any way any impressions that the community consultations have a significance that they do not have. The reasons policy-makers are seeking community consultations can be openly shared with participants. It is not necessarily true that community members will refuse an invitation to participate if the researcher explains that there is no guarantee that their views about policy solutions will be used because, for example, the exercise is more about exploring a range of possible options. It may be enough for community members to know that the researcher is an 'honest broker' who will clearly and impartially document their views in the report for policy-makers. Regardless of popular stereotypes of the naïveté of community members, few these days assume that their views will shape policy in any direct or simple way.

Recommended reading

Minkler M, Wallerstein N, (Eds). *Community Based Participatory Research for Health.* San Francisco, Jossey-Bass, 2003.

Case study in consensus-building for health policy

Case study: Finding out what people want from health and social care services in the United Kingdom

The report *Our Health, Our Care, Our Say*[237] was published in 2006 as a white paper by Britain's NHS that set out directions for how health and social care services could work in partnership to better meet the needs of the British people. It is based on extensive community consultations using diverse methods to maximize participation:

1 Consultations on adult social care services responding to the specific questions envisioned in the green paper *Independence, Well-being and Choice: Our Vision for the Future of Social care for Adults in England*[238]: these consultations involved 1,511 submissions and 2,000 people participating in regional and national consultation events, with a composite total of 100,000 people being involved often via their organizational involvement and regional organizational consultation.[239]

2 Consultations on how health and social care services can work together involving 40,000 people: a core questionnaire (29,808 people); magazine surveys (3,358 people); local listening exercises or community meetings (8,468 people); regional deliberative events (254 people); national citizens' summit.[237]

The consultations for social care services were run by an independent agency working in collaboration with the Department of Health. They emphasized gathering data from service users, especially those whose views were not so well-represented. This involved commissioning specialists to help facilitate the participation of these groups, for example, by way of developing 'easy read' versions of the consultation materials. Twenty-eight percent of all community submissions received on adult social care were in these easy-to-read formats. Summaries of the green paper were prepared in six different languages, as well as in Braille and audio formats. A consultation toolkit was developed for use in focus groups.[239]

The analysis of the data on social care involved defining key areas of interest: direct payments and individual budgets; prevention; risk management; service vision; and assessment. The reporting of the results of consultations followed the structure of the green paper so that readers could see the results of the consultations under the headings defined in the green paper. The nature and strength of community feeling about different categories of responses to different aspects of the green paper's proposals were presented in bar carts, pie graphs, and in tables, as well as discussion in the main text using summary percentages. Bar charts and line graphs offer details of key aspects of the findings of the consultations (such as 'top prevention ideas from the consultations' p. 46) as well as related population data collected by the project to support the policy arguments being made. Shaded boxes were used to capture quotations from community participants. Boxes were also used to highlight the data about 'what works' in health reform and showcase key aspects of government policy and principles for reform. The report included case studies of exemplar local service approaches to certain health challenges such as improving mental health. The case studies were also used to offer vignettes of particular health challenges that were overcome by individuals participating in the consultations, such as the story of Gary Buchner's efforts to lose weight and become fit with his peer group in the Braunstone housing estate in Leicester. Summary sections under each of the headings were used to highlight the 'take home' messages of the consultations.[239]

In this way the design and analysis of the consultations was a cohesive part of a larger set of research investigations and policy arguments in *Our Health, Our Care, Our Say*.[237] More than that, the report suggests the diverse ways in which the voice of communities may be represented in a report for health policy: with different research methods, different ways of collecting, analysing, and presenting data, different typographical features of the report, and so on.

Chapter 7

Telling the health policy story

Overview

The chapter describes and offers practical strategies for the art of delivering written policy arguments. Chapters 1 to 6 dealt with how to decipher the policy problem, as well as design and analyse research that speaks to the policy problem. This chapter analyses techniques for writing the report in a way that delivers the policy story, from understanding the nature of political reasoning in policy-making contexts to special issues in data presentation for policy-makers. It emphasizes that delivering findings in this genre is not just about research rigour—it is about particular strategic written communication skills.

The policy story defined

> This concept of stories is always so important in getting people to listen. Those are the kinds of things that I'm thinking of when we're trying to influence the health system using a new piece of information. How you create a compelling story that allows you to attract attention to the outcome of the research? Usually it has a patient attached to it.

> (health agency CEO)

The art of translating research into a persuasive argument for policy options is the art of telling the policy story. There is no doubt that the definition of the policy problem and its solutions involves a form of story-telling; that policy analysis is in part a creative art.[155] The challenge for researchers for policy-making is not to eliminate policy stories in the interests of a seeming objectivity, but rather to become masters of that story-telling craft.

The policy story is a particular kind of narrative that requires its own set of knowledge and skills. It is constructed from the mosaic of formal and informal evidence to speak to the policy problem. However, the policy story does not focus only on generalizable effect sizes since its aim is to engage with a specific policy context. Instead, the researcher attempts to synthesize policy findings to create a policy story that involves high-level quali-quantitative analytic,

strategic, political and conceptual skills to bring together a 'mixed bag' of
vidence about a local policy problem. This involves:

- accurately deciphering the policy context in a situation in which that context can only ever be imperfectly read, including with social practices of
fact-finding such as negotiation and networking to uncover the unwritten
arguments that may work in that policy context

- analysing the data in policy-relevant ways that reflect good judgments about
policy reasoning i.e. the nature of the evidence, empirical and normative,
required for a policy argument

- telling the policy story in ways informed by an awareness of strategic-political
language issues to do with community and media reception of the report.

Key ideas

Accordingly, the policy story can be defined as the synthesis of evidence
provided by the researcher into a policy argument. Such arguments use
distinctive styles of reasoning, outlined in this chapter, to offer solutions to
the explicit and implicit elements of the policy problem.

As the chapter on deciphering the policy problem suggested, the definition
of the policy problem is often the result of a struggle between opposing interests and groups. Such competing policy stories can be captured through community-based research explored in Chapter 6. Policy analysts rightly argue that
those who produce and control the interpretation of the policy problem also
have considerable power to control how solutions to the policy problem are
made.[74] The policy story is often adversarial in the sense that it writes back
against these competing explanations of the policy problem, seeking to assert
its own definition of the policy problem, as well as the causes and solutions. In
a sense, the policy story is often a detailed argument for preferring a particular
definition of the policy problem and its causes and solutions.

The enabling assumptions of policy stories

The previous section suggested that policy-making is, in part, a struggle
between different kinds of stories that represent different kinds of values.[155]
Each of these stories is suggestive of a particular course of action policy-
makers should take. The art of policy story-telling involves an awareness of these
competing policy stories and a capacity to write back against their enabling
assumptions.

Key ideas

The 'enabling assumption' of a policy story is the single or related (and sometimes contradictory) set of assumptions upon which the policy story relies for its veracity.

For example, a policy story in the media about the value of residential care of adolescents with substance abuse issues may rely on the assumption that this service setting really does deliver better outcomes than other service settings (hospital outpatient settings, at-home and youth outreach 'street-level' services and so on).

A 'health myth' is a policy story that is based on wrong or unsubstantiated enabling assumptions. For example, unless the myth that residential services always deliver the best outcomes is examined with empirical evidence astutely synthesized into a counter policy argument, it may be difficult to get policy about adolescent substance abuse reoriented to at-home service modes. This may be because representatives of community services, consumers, and youth health practitioners continue to insist that a residential service is what's needed in that community.

The enabling assumptions of competing policy arguments can take many forms. Accounts of real world policy-making produced by the UK Cabinet Office emphasize that failed policy is often based on unexamined assumptions, whether they are about how people behave, how computers work, or how systems operate.[18] Accordingly, the work of telling the policy story is about more than simply putting forward evidence supporting a particular policy option. It is about deciphering and writing back against the very diverse ways in which assumptions can lead to errors of policy-making.

Of course, enabling assumptions in policy stories are sometimes right, or partly right, or right at some level or in some way for some group. Yet even when a competing policy story implying or advocating a course of action relies on an enabling assumption that is absolutely right, there may be another better option. The better option may rely on an assumption that is equally right. This is because an enabling assumption is not the singular element that makes a policy story and its implicit or explicit option right for a particular community. It is simply an assumption.

The value-laden nature of policy story-telling

Any advice on policy story-telling that neglects the ways in which that story belongs to a political struggle over values would have limited its value for researchers 'out in the field.' As Deborah Stone has argued in *The Policy Paradox*,[155] research for policy has engaged with at least two different and often warring concepts of society: the market model and the polis model. The market model of society involves a focus on competitive individual interests and achievement as the basis of decision-making and change. The polis model involves a focus on trying to balance self-interest against community interest through cooperation and competition as the building blocks of decision-making and change.[155] Much of the language of health policy stories can be understood in terms of a tension between these different values.

Reasoning and persuading in policy story-telling

Persuasion is important to policy-making because many policy constraints cannot be changed without also changing values and opinions.[71] The role of policy arguments is thus to give acceptable reasons for policy choices.[71] Policy story-telling is also about using a whole range of techniques for reasoning and persuading, including

- arguments about policy goals such as equity and equality, efficiency (including market efficiency), and equality-efficiency trade-offs, security (and security-efficiency trade-offs), liberty (and liberty-security trade-offs)
- notions of empirical causality (in scholarly evidence), as well as other notions of causality
- arguments about the public interest
- inducements and rules
- facts
- arguments about normative rights and beliefs
- strategic use of language, number, typographical, and unwritten symbols.

Each of these is examined in turn in the pages that follow.

Key ideas

This chapter suggests that the nature of the policy argument is often dialectical: when empirical data are not available, it may be enough that the premises of the argument are plausible and present in the community, for example, in relation to health services issues about which there is strong consensus. This means the argument may not always involve a formal proof as in scientific writing but rather a shared understanding of the policy issues.[71]

As Majone concludes in *Evidence, Argument and Persuasion in the Policy Process*

> Good policy analysis is more than data analysis or a modelling exercise; it also provides standards of argument and an intellectual structure for public discourse. Even when its conclusions are not accepted, its categories and language, its criticism of traditional approaches, and its advocacy of new ideas affect—even condition—the policy debate.[71] (p. 7)

The goals of policy in story-telling

Identifying the archetypal goals of policy can help better understand generic techniques of persuasion in policy story-telling. This section discusses different kinds of archetypal goals in policy arguments and the story-telling styles associated with them in ways that build upon and bring a health policy focus to the work of Stone in her book *The Policy Paradox*.

Key ideas

The particular archetypal goals of policy arguments to be considered from Stone's work are: equity and equality, efficiency (including market efficiency), and equality-efficiency trade-offs, security (and security-efficiency trade-offs), liberty (and liberty-security trade-offs).[155] Examples of these kinds of policy arguments for health policy are also given.

Concepts of equality relate to ideas about how each member of a society should or can have the same share of resources,[155] whether they are intangible resources such as access to quality services, or material resources such as bricks and mortar. As a goal, equality presents many complex policy issues and dilemmas. For example, policy-makers must decide who will be the recipients of the resources to be divided, what will be divided, and how it will be divided.[155] People are not equal in society hence resources will need to be often divided unequally to achieve a more level playing field. For example, the goal that health outcomes should be equal involves making complex decisions about which members of a society need to be targeted using what resources in what ways.

Efficiency can be understood as being about getting the best possible output for a given input. This involves complex decisions about what are the correct outputs and objectives, and who should benefit from these outputs, as well as decisions about what and how inputs should be counted, including the opportunity costs of using an input in one way rather than another.[155] In complex democratic market economies, many things can shape efficiency, from market imperfections to the realities of how communities work.[155]

For example, the goal of efficiency in a particular hospital involves decisions about what the objectives of a hospital should be (ensure short waiting times for essential surgery and so on) who the hospital should serve (its local community or people from a larger region), and what should be counted as hospital inputs, how (direct government funding, existing and new material capital equipment, staffing, positive changes in the region that attract better quality staff, and so on). The efficiency of that hospital may be affected by a broad range of factors from the rising costs of health insurance caused by the dominance of a few insurers to the influx of older persons with chronic conditions into the region.

Arguments that to have efficiency one must sacrifice equality and vice versa are themselves very value-laden. For example, it could be argued that a hospital cannot be located in a rural area because it will be impossible to attract the specialist staff required for efficient service delivery. Stone argues that the efficiency and equality are not mutually exclusive, but she does not present systematic evidence that this is so in a book in which she makes her support for a polis-driven vision of society very clear.[155] It seems likely that sometimes there will be hard policy choices to make between equality and efficiency. Clearly, evidence-based policy research should not create the illusion that equality must be sacrificed in the interests of efficiency when innovative problem-solving can show the two goals are achievable.

Many arguments in health policy revolve around concepts of need. This includes considerations of how to decide and value resources to meet particular needs, how the allocation of resources compares across different groups and systems, what should be the agreed-upon purposes of resources, how much and what kinds of forward planning to meet health needs should be done, and so on.[155] For example, assessment of chronic disease prevention needs for particular groups defined by chronic disease (or a combination of such conditions) would most likely involve consideration of needs based on questions about what resources should be given to which groups in what ways for what length of time. This is likely to be so in a context in which the evidence may indicate that some groups more than others already have well-developed advocacy groups that have provided particular kinds of assistance through services such as information and training sessions, counselling and support groups. The fact that needs are dynamic over time and heterogeneous across different groups and individuals adds complexity to policy arguments.

Put simply, security relates to the extent to which the needs of an individual or group are met.[155] There will be different standards held by different groups for what is an acceptable level for meeting health needs. Universal health coverage is one such standard. For example, some societies such as Britain have achieved greater consensus that health is a right and not a privilege to be purchased. In other societies such as America, history, culture and economics have interacted to make universal health cover an elusive goal. Policy arguments can be made for and against government involvement in securing greater or lesser health coverage for particular items such as oral healthcare or emergency medical services for the general society and for particular groups such as older people or children, or people with disabilities. Thus security or the extent to which needs can be met is a policy goal that is very much defined by policy argument.

In some contexts there will be possibilities for achieving security and efficiency without compromising either. In other contexts this will not be possible. Again, ideally an evidence-based policy argument will provide innovative problem-solving that helps policy-makers achieve the two goals to the maximum extent possible.

Liberty is another policy goal explored by Stone which she defines as the freedom to do as one wishes unless that affects the rights of others.[155] This policy goal can involve quite complex considerations to do with deciding the nature of harms to others that should lead to government restraints on the liberties of individuals, groups or organizations, and whose liberty should be restrained in what way.[155] For example, in health policy at the individual and group level there can be some quite complex arguments about the nature of interventions for people with particular mental health conditions that may lead them to harm others. At the organizational level there can be complex arguments that private health insurance companies ought not be self-regulating because their right to pursue free market goals leading to ever greater dominance of fewer and fewer companies interferes with the rights of others to enjoy affordable health insurance.

Again, there are arguments that liberty and security can co-exist as policy goals, as well as arguments that they are incompatible goals.[155] For example, it could be argued that free universal healthcare cover is important because the security of this cover actually works to liberate citizens. Yet there will be some who argue that in fact it offers a case in point of how incompatible the two goals are because free coverage can only be bought by imposing greater taxes on a portion of the population. Ideally, evidence-based policy arguments will demonstrate that needs can be met without sacrificing the liberty of citizens.

There are also arguments that liberty and equality can co-exist as policy goals, and contrary arguments that having one means sacrificing the other.[155] For example, arguments that rural communities need to have more equal numbers of general practitioners can be accompanied by the view that overseas doctors should be bonded by the terms of their visas to work in more isolated areas. Yet one could make a policy argument that too great restrictions on such doctors and their families (a 10 year versus a 5 year bond?) is exploitative and irreconcilable with basic standards of freedom and the duty of care that a society owes to immigrant workers.

Using causality in policy story-telling

As Chapters 4 and 5 suggested, different research methods are based on different ideas about causality. Technical debates about causality among quantitative researchers will be different from debates about causality among qualitative researchers. As this book has also suggested, what matters for policy-making is the extent to which research can accurately capture causal complexity in ways that are useful to multidisciplinary, high stakes policy decision-making.

However, causality can also be understood as an element of the art of policy story-telling. This is because persuasive research for policy is about more than accuracy. It is also about using 'causal stories' strategically.

Key practical strategy

Explanations of causality can be used to

◆ analyse the policy problem and assign responsibility for the cause of the problem

◆ debunk policy myths and challenge the assumptions informing particular interests and practices

◆ argue against counter proposals and pre-empt criticism of the preferred policy options

◆ support preferred policy options and buttress the role of particular organizations in helping solve the policy problem.[155]

In relation to the last point, understandings of the cause of the policy problem can be used to shape how policy-makers and their communities understand the policy solutions. Thus definitions of policy problems also need to be understood as 'strategic representations' that control and regulate policy meanings in order to affirm a particular course of action.[155, 240, 241]

For example, applying Stone's argument[242] to the contexts of health policy, research for health policy could explain the policy problem of a hospital closure in terms of accident (the hospital never recovered from cyclone damage), the agency of individuals (staff morale declined after the appointment of a new CEO), secret intentions of the government (economic rationalist approaches to small rural hospitals), risk-taking behaviours by the government (cost-cutting not intended to lead to the hospital's closure), or a broader divide between rural and urban areas that has created disadvantage in many areas of essential services.

In summary, whatever else it is, policy story-telling is about weaving a cohesive narrative about the cause of the policy problem.

A tool for making arguments about public interests

Arguments about the public interest can have great persuasive power in health policy research. Policy arguments that do not account for all the relevant interests may be more likely to fail. Stone offers a list of concepts of interests[155] that have been developed in this book to apply to the contexts of health policy. The way in which interests are felt and perceived is critical to public interest arguments. In health policy, interests can be subjectively felt by different individuals and groups or they can exist independent of the awareness of particular groups.

Subjectively felt interests could relate to those healthcare phenomena, practical arrangements, policies, and so on that people perceive as affecting them.[155] For example, when a mental health advocacy group voices its concerns about the lack of funding for mental health it may describe the effects of this on children. Such perceptions can exist independently of whether the phenomena under question are actually affecting groups and individuals.

Objectively felt interests relate to those healthcare phenomena, practical arrangements, policies, and so on that affect groups without their awareness of those effects. For example, population health data may show a previously unknown link between low iodine levels in childhood and cognitive functioning in a particular demographic area.

The task of research for health policy is thus often to present evidence that demonstrates how particular public interests may best be served, in contexts in which the interests themselves may need to be defined by the research. In making a policy argument that includes arguments about the public interest it can be helpful to develop a map, based on the results of research, about the different kinds of interests that may be involved. Table 7.1 offers some examples of different kinds of interests often found in health and the challenges of defining and arguing for those interests. It is not meant to be all-encompassing (not all interests are defined by groups), but rather to illustrate the diversity of interests in health that researchers may need to consider. These will not be static, such that often researchers are offering policy arguments about interests that may develop in the future. The table can be used as a tool for auditing policy arguments to see if they do adequately account for the different interests.

Table 7.1 Examples of interests

Type of interest group	Challenges in defining and arguing for such interests
Professional organizations	May not represent all members of the profession: multiple professional organizations can have different competing interests
Private healthcare sector	Often competing commercial interests with some shared interests
Non-government sector	May be competing for limited healthcare funding and market share; likely to be defined by diverse organizational missions, cultures and practices
Government	Political and bureaucratic interests define different departments and units within departments, as well as individuals and groups defined by level of seniority and role within the government healthcare bureaucracy (for example, practitioners versus management)
Politicians	Likely to represent different party policies and ideologies that are themselves not homogenous, and be defined by different short-term and long-term interests and pressures
Patients	Interests will be different depending on health condition, culture, socio-economic status, age, geographical location, and so on; patient advocacy groups likely to reflect diverse and conflicting perspectives

Public interest arguments therefore involve defining which interests are affected, and which interests should be served by particular policy options. Many of the research methods and approaches described in this book, such as in Chapter 6 on consensus-building for health policy, are designed to assist in delivering evidence that accounts for such interests.

Of course, arguments about the public interest present extraordinarily complex strategic, political, and ethical dilemmas. Public interest arguments can involve considerable manipulation: for example, making particular policy options seem less deleterious for some groups than they actually are, or arguing that a wide range of interests will be served by an option that is actually serving only very narrow interests. These kinds of manipulations are unethical because they involve distorting the truth (as far as it can be understood by the available evidence). Inevitably any policy option will serve one set of interests more than another. From one perspective, policy argument has a place in ethical research insofar as it helps researchers make the evidence about interests more transparent, including the hard decisions that need to be made about which interests should be served.

Inducements, rules and rights

Stone[155] describes policy argument also in terms of inducements. Inducements can be used in policy arguments to persuade particular groups of the value of policy options. For example, the allocation of resources such as funding and health service benefits to particular groups can work to persuade them of the value of particular policy options. These can involve quite complex issues: for example, the meaning of the inducement to the target group may be quite different from what is intended by the researcher and/or the inducement may be dismissed as a cheap tactic to win support for the policy option. The use of inducements should be based on careful research and strategic thinking: inducements are ideally founded on consensus-building approaches such as those described in Chapter 6.

Stone also discusses the importance of rules in policy arguments.[155] Some policy arguments have failed because they have violated a particular written or unwritten rule or code. Health research is necessarily hemmed in by a broad range of legislative and regulatory requirements that form part of the policy argument for particular options. There are also many unwritten protocols that can shape arguments for health policy, such as an unwritten rule that a particular powerful group be allowed to self-regulate. Such rules can work powerfully within a sector such as health precisely because they are unwritten. These written and unwritten rules may explicitly and implicitly inform the policy argument. Some researchers can be very skilled in using particular forms of evidence about rules, such as legislation, to develop strong policy arguments.

Arguments about human rights in health policy can also be used to create powerful policy stories. Stone[155] defines four kinds of rights which are explained here with reference to health systems:

- procedural rights or the right to have decisions made according to a particular process such as the rights of patients to make complaints to a medical board
- substantive rights or rights to claim a specific entitlement or action such as the right to emergency department health services regardless of income
- negative rights or rights to do something without being prevented by others such as the right to refuse medical treatment
- positive rights or rights to hold or be given something such as the right to be given tax subsidized prescription medicines if you are over a certain age.

Researchers for policy will therefore need to be aware of the complex web of rights that are defined in statutes, rules and regulations, and related precedence and the mechanisms by which those rights are exercised and enforced.[155]

A tool for using facts in policy arguments

I like the colourful fact that we all can rally around and try to figure out how to address, you know, what's the number one killer, those kind of things, but for other people it is the story that galvanizes action.

(health agency CEO)

A fact is an apparently undeniable phenomenon. Yet as Chapter 1 suggested, there are many other things besides facts that can work to shape health policy decision-making. In a policy world of political spin, facts can be highly interpretative and information may be more about achieving a desired effect than truth-telling. However, it is not as if the only choice is between telling the truth as such and being Machiavellian. In practice there are many other kinds of choices to be made about how the presentation of facts will shape perceptions. Researchers for policy may spend much time reflecting on and gathering information about how, for example, different groups and individuals may read different and equally truthful ways of presenting the same factual information. The approaches to community consensus-building described in Chapter 6 should help establish what those different meanings are among different stakeholders. Using the work of Stone[155] as a point of departure, Table 7.2 is designed to help illustrate the range of different kinds of facts and challenges in using them in policy arguments. It can be used as a tool to help researchers reflect on whether they are using different kinds of facts effectively in their reports to make sound policy arguments.

Table 7.2 Examples of facts

Kind of fact	Example	Challenges in using such facts in policy arguments
Fact about community opinion or belief	That most people believe healthcare cover should be universal for all children	Such facts may be dependent on context and highly conditional; they may also be irrelevant if narrow interests are more powerful
Rule-based fact	That in 2008 the United States Congress passed the 'Veterans Health Care Budget Reform Act', which aims to provide arrangements that help Congress ensure sufficient funding levels for veterans' healthcare	Such facts may be problematic given that the intention of rules may be at odds with their effects, and when implemented rules are often subverted by different interests
Fact about material resources	The EEG recorder in the Neurosurgery unit needs upgrading	The nature and adequacy of material resources can be highly contentious
Fact about funding	That the national budget delivered the government's commitment for $1.9 billion to improve services for people with a mental illness	The meaning of funding is highly relative and dependent on a wide range of contextual financial and other factors
Bio-scientific fact	The mutation rate in the human genome is about twice as high in male as in female meiosis	The implications of bio-scientific facts for policy and practice are often unclear and subject to dispute as well as qualification by later scientific research

Table 7.2 (continued) Examples of facts

Kind of fact	Example	Challenges in using such facts in policy arguments
Statistical fact	75% of all respondents in the chronic disease self-management study indicated they had school leaving or higher qualifications. However, lower education levels were positively related to non-completion of the programme	The implications of statistical facts may be too general to be helpful to the specifics of the local contextual policy problem. Such facts often have to be carefully assembled to make a cohesive policy story
Fact about causal conditions	Medication errors have caused the majority of adverse events at the local hospital	Facts about causal conditions can be true at one level but disguise the deeper underlying causal effects that need to be known before a policy solution can be found

The following section on sign systems is designed to explore the possibilities for strategic representation of information, including known facts, in the policy argument.

Using sign systems in policy story-telling

The legislature and the governor are inundated with research, they're inundated with papers, they're inundated with things that they need to read to understand more fully what's going on . . . most of the time if they feel that the research is sound they go with it. And what makes them have a confidence in the research probably depends on where the research comes from, the credibility of the researcher themselves—in other words maybe Harvard would be more credible than the University of Bermuda or something. If the research is done by somebody they know—which doesn't happen very often—that enhances the credibility. Probably who financed the research is incredibly important, particularly in medicine and drug company studies etc. And quite honestly how the research is presented, if it's really good research and it's presented in a very easy to read and understandable manner I think it's much more credible and understood than if it comes across as a bunch of jargon that's very difficult to read and understand.

(health agency CEO)

This section considers in turn each of the different sign systems used in policy story-telling, and techniques for using these signs to create powerful and credible policy stories:

- language symbols: stories, anecdotes and synecdoches, metaphors, and the use of ambiguity and subtexts
- number sign systems: the use of numbers as metaphors, norms, symbols, and so on in story-telling for policy-makers and the wider community.

There are, of course, other sign systems worthy of consideration. For example, typographical sign systems: the use of typographical features of the text to tell the policy story, including the use of presentation forms that allow for different levels of information giving and rapid scanning of the evidence[81] These have been highlighted in some of the case studies presented in this book. As Chapter 6 has also suggested, there are also unwritten sign systems: the production of meaning in, for example, public personas important to the performative aspects of policy-relevant research. In keeping with the focus of this chapter on developing written skills of policy argument, this chapter focuses on the two main sign systems involved—language and numbers.

Using language symbols

> . . . backing up the data-driven description that has the evidentiary basis with a simple story about what this actually means is a time honoured technique that we constantly use. So to say 'This intervention has been effective in changing the outcome of this particular disease and here's a graph that demonstrates a four year improvement in survival as an example' is a good way to tell the story. But an even better way, or to add to that story is to say, 'And here's a patient who been in that situation, here's what this patient was experiencing, and here's what would happen if that patient was treated with intervention A. Here's what we've traditionally done for this patient. Here's the likely outcome now if intervention B was' . . . you can imagine the story that we can tell. And that story is a good story; those stories work.
>
> (health agency CEO)

Stone identifies a number of language devices that can operate symbolically in policy story-telling in a community and which have been adapted and elaborated here to make her categories more relevant to health policy:

- *archetypal narratives* which are stereotypical ways in which reality can be understood, for example, stories of decline (the story of decline of a health service or system) or stories of progress (advances in medical technology)

- *anecdote* which is about using a short colourful narrative or vignette about concrete events that may be amusing, thought-provoking or colourful: it can be used to dramatize, for example, the problems of access to a health service a particular group may be experiencing

- *synecdoche* which is a rhetorical device in which a part can be used to represent a whole (a horror hospital error story to represent the decline of the entire health system) and vice versa (the whole for a part, for example, when a horror hospital error story is used to represent the arguable lack of accountability of medical quality assurance for overseas trained doctors); the species for the genus (such as referring to the problem of hospital error in terms of overseas-trained doctors when the issue may be more a function of overworked hospital medical staff generally), the genus for the species

(suggesting the issue is about lack of medical accountability when it relates to lack of proper training of some groups of overseas-trained doctors)

- *metaphor* which is a rhetorical device for asserting likeness between one kind of thing and another (using the term 'aristocratic specialists' to suggest that specialists have certain attributes)

- *ambiguity* which is about using language to give statements more than one meaning, for example, relating the closure of a hospital in ways that suggest it is less about service closure and more about a government's unwillingness to fund rural hospitals.[155]

Each of these devices are potentially very powerful in research for policy because of their strategic value in policy story-telling. For example, anecdotes can be very useful devices in dramatizing political positions, as in Al Gore's tale of the same drug costing less for his dog than for his mother-in-law.[243] The value of anecdotal story-telling is that it helps those who hold different values in a policy dispute gain a better understanding of those value differences.

Anecdotal information also offers a language in which the research evidence can be understood: anecdotes can personalize, illustrate, and help persuade others by offering a language that is more meaningful from that used in formal research.[243, 244] Anecdotal policy stories can help explore the multidimensional nature of policy problems, client experiences, and political impacts of policy decisions that might otherwise only be communicable in the abstract. The prevalence of policy anecdotes in policy story-telling suggests how research for policy draws not simply on empirical evidence, but also the visceral and emotional dimensions of human sensibility to communicate and persuade.

In research for health policy, the anecdotes of community stakeholders can have a particularly important role to play in conveying their experience of, and views about, healthcare. For example, researchers can quote anecdotal information obtained from disadvantaged minority client groups to illuminate a finding about their service use that is reported in quantitative data. The policy story can be particularly powerful when both formal research evidence and anecdotal information appear to be mutually reinforcing. When empirical research evidence and anecdotal information are different, there will be a need to engage with this difference. This is particularly so when anecdotal information has a high street level currency that expresses the values held by a community. Anecdotal stories can be particularly useful in helping the researcher identify and 'write back' against health myths, including when presenting in community forums.

Key ideas

Each of these and other rhetorical devices can be used to persuade and reason with the audience for the policy argument: policy-makers, stakeholders, the media, and so on. The number of rhetorical devices available in language as a sign system is limited only by the policy researcher's skill and dexterity with strategic language use. What matters in evidence-based policy-making is not simply the rigor of the evidence but the extent to which researchers have engaged with the logic of pros and cons for particular policy positions. Delivering the health policy argument involves strategic representation using different kinds of language devices to reason politically.

Number symbols

Dr Foster shocked the NHS by putting out data forms for the public about what was happening to their healthcare system. The public system has moved to using those forms for presenting back within its own management. So, once you would have gone to a management committee and you'd have sat down with reams of tables and charts and words, and you wouldn't have got very many questions—a typical board meeting would have been an example of that. And that's because everybody was so far up their own backsides thinking they knew everything about everything, you didn't actually realise they didn't understand any of it at all, and were oblivious to it. But Dr Foster started to churn out in the *Sunday Times* things that were in an easy readable format that people could look at and say, 'Wow, is that really what's happening in my hospital? Is that really what the health system is doing?' And then a sea-change took place . . .

(health agency CEO)

The ability to accurately, meaningfully, and strategically use number sign symbols is a critical skill in policy story-telling and policy reasoning.

As Stone has argued, numbers are highly political.[155] This is because the use of quantitative data requires value-laden decisions about what and how to categorize—inclusion and exclusion. The measurement of any quality does involve norms and expectations. Much political struggle can take place around the interpretation of numbers which have a story-telling function. Numbers can also be used to create illusions for political purposes, for example, by simplifying a complex entity such as health service performance. Numbers can also create a new kind of reality, such as a health needs groups identified by particular ways of categorizing data. Numerical data can also work as a tool for policy-makers to negotiate solutions and compromise, through offering evidence about, for example, the history of budget allocations for healthcare services.[155] In short, number sign systems as much as language sign systems offer many ways of strategically using meaning to help diagnose the policy problem and suggest solutions. Porter has argued in his famous book *Trust in Numbers: The Pursuit of Objectivity in Science and Public Life* that numbers have acquired a seeming objectivity that has given them unprecedented authority in public policy-making.[242]

The definitive work on making quantitative data meaningful for the wider community, including policy-makers is the 2009 book *Making Data Talk: The Science and Practice of Translating Public Health Research and Surveillance Findings to Policy Makers, the Public, and the Press* by Nelson, Hess, and Croyle.[73] This book suggests the importance of not just numbers, but also weaving numbers and words together in making sound policy arguments.

Key practical strategy

The work of Nelson, Hess, and Croyle[73] provides the basis for the following practical advice in using numbers to tell a story:

1 *Make sound, parsimonious decisions about whether the data should be included in the text at all.* This may seem an obvious point, however, research for policy can suffer from the flaw that the data presented do not quite address the point at hand, however rigorous and meaningful they are for some other issue.

2 *Ensure that the policy story is exact in its interpretation of the data.* Many research reports for policy can be unpersuasive if the words used to describe data analyses do not bear an exact relationship to those data. For example, researchers need to beware of implying causality when two types of data are correlated. Where complex data analyses are involved much thought may need to be given to the accuracy of the words chosen to interpret those analyses.

3 *Carefully consider whether randomness might explain the phenomena under examination.* Research for policy will be vulnerable to criticism if it attributes causality to patterns in data that are artefacts of randomness.

4 *Make sound decisions about the 'fitness for purpose' of the quantitative analyses to be used.* This is not simply about technical judgement, it is also about making a sound judgment of the match between the data analysis method and the policy problem.

5 *Ensure that the data presented speak to the enabling assumptions and health myths that must be countered if the policy argument is to succeed.* As this

Key practical strategy *(continued)*

chapter has emphasized, good policy arguments are not just about determining what policy options are supported by the evidence. They are also about delivering evidence that can speak to assumptions and myths that will prevent evidence-based policy from succeeding.

6 *Select data analyses and supporting explanations that speak to the problems of uncertainty.* Unless data analyses do this, it is unlikely that policy arguments will succeed. The section discussing uncertainty in Chapter 2 offers a point of departure for auditing data analyses to ensure they do address all the possible issues of uncertainty.

7 *Pay attention to the likely numeracy levels of policy-makers and their communities* and make choices about what to present, how, which are influenced by this knowledge of audience. The use of typographical strategies such as technical boxes can be most helpful here. The art of offering short and accessible explanations for complex data analyses that leave nothing important out is a complex one. What often matters most is that lay policy-makers (some have high levels of technical understanding) can grasp the underlying logic of the analysis and explain it to their communities. Nelson, Hess, and Croyle offer a thorough discussion of this challenge in their book.[73]

8 *Make the connections between the findings and the decision-making context explicit.* Some reports for policy do not succeed because that connection is too abstruse. Research for policy should explain what the findings mean for the policy decisions that have to be made.[73]

The use of quantitative data in health policy story-telling is also limited only by the researcher's skill and imagination. For example, recent years have seen a number of important developments in the art of using spatial statistics to tell policy stories. There are models of how to use 'small area comparisons' to offer better consideration of regional variations involving smaller geographical areas than traditional analyses directed at provinces, states, or country level data.[245] Small area comparisons have value for policy-making because they target the contexts that may be most relevant to local area decision-making. They can do so using visual representations of data (coloured maps) that allow a large amount of data to be conveyed economically. However, such methods also suffer from well-known problems of accuracy of the population information of these small areas.[245]

Approaches to representing regional differences using spatial statistics can range from simple representations of socio-economic differences between regions to visual representations of differences in the views of community members in different regions included in community consensus-making exercises.[245] By doing so small area comparisons can, in a single picture, point to policy arguments that need to be argued for or against. For example, small area mapping can be used to show that while prevailing policy arguments rely on the assumption that poverty in rural communities is linked to poor health outcomes, this cannot explain what is happening in particular small rural areas relevant to the local policy context.[245]

However sophisticated the scholarly literature, policy-makers often emphasize the importance of 'keeping it simple, stupid':

> . . . in the areas where I have an influence on policy, which is usually in a committee meeting room or whatever, the important thing is to have the background of the research and be able to verbalize it in a very simple, very concise, very short dialogue that drives home a point . . . if you bring up more than one or two points I think from that point on you're probably not going to be successful . . . if you start showing data and graphs—people very rarely explain a graph very well, they very rarely go into the x axis or the y axis or explain the bar—people get lost and their eyes get glazed over. And then the problem is that your credibility drops off very rapidly and people just quit listening.
>
> (health agency CEO)

Communicating complex data in ways that are accessible to laypersons is not easy to accomplish. Nelson, Hess, and Croyle offer a discussion of the literature explaining, for example, how people visually process graphs and other images, useful to researchers who need to make decisions about where to position such material in their reports. They also offer many 'dos and don'ts' for many different ways of visually presenting numerical data.[73] Ideally, researchers will work with editors and other typographical experts to ensure that they have maximized the possibilities for persuading and explaining in the presentation of their data. This will involve ethical considerations:

> . . . it's important that presentations—especially when they are being provided to lay groups who don't necessarily have the background of interpretation of statistical data—are presented in ethical ways. That's the baseline of where I think we need to start: the ethical decision, the ethical presentation of data in a way that's understandable. Also, you shouldn't take advantage of other groups in presenting with data in a way that wouldn't be acceptable to a truly sophisticated scientific audience.
>
> At the same time, you do need to take advantage of the types of graphics or the types of presentations, to make them more straightforward and understandable . . . You shouldn't have to work hard at a graph to understand it.
>
> (health agency CEO)

The implied policy-maker

The importance of the implied policy-maker has received little attention in scholarly policy studies. However, the idea that every text has an implied reader is common to literary analysis, and in particular reader-response theory.[246] The way an individual writes suggests an image of how that individual imagines the reader. Writing voice operates at that powerful visceral and aesthetic level that makes a reader say 'I want to be the person this writer imagines I am.' Some of United States president Barack Obama's power as a public speaker and consensus-maker appears to relate to his ability to create the altruistic and principled self people want to be. Skilled policy-making researchers carefully modulate the tone, style, and manner of their writing—their writing voice—to create an implied reader that is attractive to policy-makers.

A key aspect of the policy-maker implied by the genre of policy-relevant research is the idea that this is an astute person who is capable of appreciating complex ideas telescoped into as few words as possible. The generic voice of policy-relevant research reflects the art of compression. Strunk and White's book *The Elements of Style* rightly emphasizes that such compression characterizes reader-friendly non-fiction styles.[247] However, in policy-relevant research, this art of compression is particularly important for accurately creating the implied reader. There is no unnecessary repetition in the best policy-relevant research reports. There is helpful restatement and elaboration of critical ideas and findings at strategic points for the advancement of policy problem-solving. Policy-relevant research is highly structured and directed, marshalling knowledge and evidence in ways that suggest not simply that strategic 'story-telling' is happening, but also that policy-makers are a particular kind of knowledge consumer. That is, they are consumers of knowledge not given for its own sake (for enlightenment) but rather for the socially instrumental purposes of policy problem-solving. The implied reader of this genre is thus rather different from the implied reader of a scholarly research paper in a peer-reviewed journal.

The writing voice in this genre also aims to convey precisely the right style and amount of deference. This is critical to the unobtrusively persuasive and adversarial nature of the content. Every statement is ideally linked to evidence of some kind, not simply for the sake of scholarship but also because the policy-maker will need to tell an evidence-based story if the preferred policy options are to be accepted. In policy-making contexts, the writing voice of research often positions itself as delivering a service. Ultimately it has the ambitious aim of adding value to the policy-maker's often long history of deliberation of the policy challenge. This means it aims to speak from inside the world of policy, reflecting back to the policy-maker the 'strategic smarts' that are so valued in these contexts. The tone is often dispassionate, measured, nuanced by an understanding of policy constraints, and politically self-aware.

Thus, the voice of written evidence for policy often aims to deliver the sharp and illuminating insight at precisely the right moment to sum up the researcher's consideration of the evidence, mirroring the deliberative yet economical nature of policy reflection. The next section explores how to generate such insights using hierarchical structuring of research evidence.

Meeting the challenge of structure in policy writing

> Often you read a research paper and then you read the recommendations and it's really not clear whether or not the researcher paid any attention at all to their own findings, or if they had a point of view and just wrote that at the end . . .

> (health agency CEO)

Scholarly literature on bridging the research-policy divide has rarely focussed on detailing and understanding the particular writing styles preferred by policy-makers. This section argues that a tightly hierarchical written structure is an important part of the generic features of policy-relevant research.

The four kinds of evidence highlighted in this book—previous local, national, and international experiences, as well as present local community experience and views—are ideally presented in ways that are helpful to the policy-maker's conceptualization of the policy problems and the full range of possible policy solutions. This means the internal conceptual architecture of the written report is quite critical. A conceptual architecture that is illuminating to a community advocate wanting an introduction to the policy challenges may be disastrous for a policy-maker with high level policy problem-solving skills and a long history of reflecting on the particular policy challenges in question. Policy-makers are interested in illuminating elaborations of the policy problems and possible solutions, bringing together each of the four kinds of evidence. The headings used in the report are therefore not simply organizers or 'signposts'. They must function as tools of persuasion and inductive advancement of the policy problem-solving process being enacted by the research report. The headings and sub-headings need to be evaluated by the researcher in terms of whether they will be helpful to the *specific* policy-makers to whom the research evidence is being delivered, in line with Majone's emphasis on giving policy-makers a persuasive story.[71]

The evidence in the policy-relevant report is often ideally arranged in layers, forming a pyramid, with every part supporting the total structure. Figure 7.1 offers a simplified visualization of this conceptual structure.

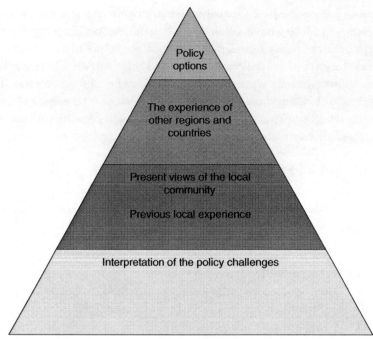

Fig. 7.1 The conceptual structure of a policy-relevant report.

In practice, as this book has suggested, the process of defining the policy challenges is iterative: for example, exploring views of the local community will refine how the policy challenges are understood.

The pyramid diagram reflects a culture of economy of words and utility of evidence noted in the last section: policy options driven by evidence that is in turn driven by interpretations of the policy problems. Policy-relevant research writing has its own style of creativity through story-telling, as this chapter has emphasized, however, that story-telling is tightly hierarchical. Structurally it is located at one end of a spectrum that has post-modernist poetry at the other. A post-modernist poem does not fulfil reader expectations of clear and explicit relationships between its different parts. The text is disordered in ways that may or may not be meaningful. Unlike the poetry reader, the policy-maker does not want to do any unnecessary work of meaning-making. Too many research reports for policy-makers fail because they are 'badly written': prolix, disorganized, and full of redundancies, instead of moving the reader systematically through a tightly orchestrated body of evidence. In policy-making 'badly written' often means the research has failed to meet such expectations of a tightly hierarchical story.

Majone has argued that distinctive methods of enquiry and ways of argumentation for policy have emerged over the history of democracy to aid the process of public deliberation.[71] The strongly hierarchical feature of policy-relevant research may have emerged historically partly in response to the complexity of evidence with which policy-makers have to engage. This book has suggested that in health the evidence in this genre must reflect the multi-dimensional nature of bio-psycho-social models of health meaningful to policy decision-makers, 'approximating complex causal patterns, and illuminating policy choices and trade-offs'.[248] Not only that, but without good unity and integration of complex evidence, distillation of the findings into the 'good story' with face-value credibility that policy-makers need becomes very difficult.[52] The policy literature suggests that one barrier to the use of research evidence by policy-makers is the lack of research skills of some policy-makers.[57] If so, policy-relevant research must be accessible to them and yet sufficiently complex to accommodate their strategic demands. Part of the way it might do this in its written form is through tightly hierarchical meaning-making.

How exactly might the hierarchical structure of meaning function in a policy-relevant research report? What does it look like?

There can be two broad levels of the hierarchy of meaning in a policy-relevant report: microstructure and macrostructure. 'Microstructure' refers to how sentences within paragraphs and paragraphs within sections are organized. 'Macrostructure' refers to how sections and larger parts of the document are organized.

At the microstructural level, policy-relevant reports can offer:

1 *Functional organising sentences at the front end of the paragraph* i.e. the first sentence of every paragraph has an analytical, insightful sentence summarizing the evidence that follows in that paragraph; the body of the paragraph is therefore an elaboration of that 'lead sentence'; the evidence within the paragraph also must have a logical order, progressing the reader's understanding of the lead sentence.

2 *A self-sufficient pathway for readers through the section using only the first sentence of every paragraph* that gives them a comprehensive grasp of the detail of the policy argument being made; that is, the reader can grasp the content of any section in the report (and indeed the whole report) just by reading the functional organizing sentences.

3 *Section summaries above groups of paragraphs* that restate in insightful ways (not simply repeat) the contents of the functional organizing sentences in that section.

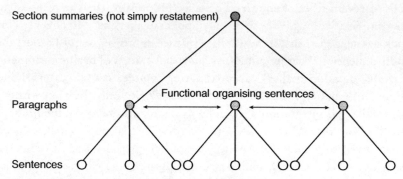

Fig. 7.2 Microstructure of a policy-relevant report.

Figure 7.2 represents this microstructure visually.

At the macrostructural level, policy-relevant reports can offer:

1 *Section summaries* giving the reader an insightful overview (not repetition) of the content of the sections (these can also be grouped into chapters that also have a summary at their front end, and the chapters can also be grouped into parts each with summaries).

2 A comprehensive but concise *statement of the policy challenges*, most often at the front end of the document i.e. the foundational logic of the evidence gathered.

3 A comprehensive but succinct statement of *the policy options* often given in full at the back end of the document i.e. the logical end point of the evidence.

4 *An executive summary* highlighting the last two, often at the front end of the document.

Figure 7.3 visually represents this macrostructure.

There are different reasons for thinking about using hierarchical ordering when writing a policy-relevant report. For example, readers of policy-relevant reports expect to see effective hierarchical ordering of recommendations in ways that communicate their relative value and nature. This expectation is suggested by the following criticism of the recommendations of the Acheson report described in the UK case study at the end of Chapter 1. The report was criticized as offering a 'shopping list' rather than a well-developed framework for change:

> Firstly, the recommendations are not presented in any hierarchy, and the key fact that inequalities in health follow closely on inequalities in wealth is underemphasised.

The hierarchy of meaning

2 – Macrostructure

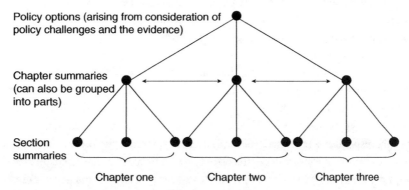

Fig. 7.3 The macrostructure of a policy-relevant report.

> The one (of 39) set of recommendations on the need to reduce poverty and income inequalities thus appears to have the same status as the recommendations on curbing traffic.[249] (p. 1465)

The writers of the Acheson report argued in reply that this criticism was wrong:

> The authors give the impression that the 39 recommendations were presented without any priority being given. In fact, we selected three clear priorities, which are the focus of our first three recommendations. These are paraphrased in the synopsis . . .[250] (p. 1659)

Whether one considers this a satisfactory reply or not, it highlights the importance of expectations that policy-relevant reports will, by virtue of distinctive hierarchical arrangements of their evidence (rather than upfront didactic instructions about intentions), *show* the reader what is important. That is, readers expect to quickly grasp the essential messages by way of effective ordering and arrangement of the material. This is not to be simply achieved by putting like things with like—though that is certainly important, as another aspect of the reply by Acheson et al. seems to suggest:

> In line with our remit to identify priority areas for policy development we assembled and assessed a large volume of evidence on each major area. It is important that each recommendation should be read in conjunction with the accompanying text. This gives a summary of the scale and nature of the inequality at which the recommendation is directed, a review of the evidence on how that inequality might be reduced, and an assessment of the expected benefit from the recommended action.[250] (p. 1659)

In fact, policy-relevant research reports offer scope for using a whole range of simple devices for signposting and reiterating messages, such as formatting headings in particular ways, offering summary boxes, and so on. As has been emphasized, the policy-relevant researcher may work closely with a graphics designer to realize the graphic-typographical possibilities for meaning-making in this genre, possibilities that are being increasingly recognized in the scholarly literature.[251] Thus, this genre of research writing can be considered as much a genre of showing as it is of telling—in this respect sharing some features of the more accessible peer-reviewed health journals that target practitioners.

There will be some who argue that including such advice about hierarchical practices of meaning-making in a book for graduates is akin to 'dumbing down' the art of researching for policy. However, as reception of the Acheson report suggests, the hierarchical ordering of evidence is an area where even highly respected senior practitioners of the art can find themselves vulnerable to criticism. The examples of this criticism with respect to the Acheson report suggest that the tightly hierarchical story-telling styles of this genre are not simply about the familiar admonishments about good structure common to undergraduate studies. They can be about quite subtle matters of evidence display. The following box offers a practical exercise readers may use as a tool for reflection on the extent to which the tight hierarchical structure diagrammed earlier is a feature of their own writing (of course, it may not need to be unless the intention is to write for policy-makers).

Practical exercise: How hierarchical is your writing?

What you will need

You will need a sample of your non-fiction writing to do this exercise. This should be at least 10 pages long so that the development of structure in your writing can be examined. Ideally, it will be a piece of research that you hope to use to change policy. However, for the purposes of this exercise it can be in any non-fiction genre: an academic essay, a briefing paper for your supervisor at work, an evaluation report, a social commentary, a grant application etc.

You will also need two highlighter pens of different colours (say, pink and green).

What to do

Step one: Take the pink highlighter pen and highlight the first sentence of every paragraph.

Step two: Take the green highlighter pen and highlight any words in your piece of writing that *best* summarize the whole argument, wherever you can find these words.

> **Practical exercise: How hierarchical is your writing?** *(continued)*
>
> Step three: Read only the words you have highlighted in pink.
>
> Step four: Read only the words you have highlighted in green.
>
> ## Reflection
>
> When you look at the content of paragraphs and audit them against the words at the front end of every paragraph (the pink words), is there a good relationship between the two?
>
> Where are the words summarizing your piece of writing (green words)? Are they all over the place or are they neatly positioned where they should be?
>
> Does your argument progress in a logical linear fashion from the beginning to the end of your piece? Or is the progress of your argument somewhat more fragmentary and halting? In other words—does your writing suggest a tight hierarchical structure?
>
> What other habits to do with the structuring of your writing do you see?

The hierarchical nature of policy-relevant research has most likely evolved in response to not simply the challenges of getting better reader comprehension in policy-making contexts. It may also be about overcoming particular writing challenges associated with those contexts. As Chapter 8 on designing policy options suggests, policy-relevant researchers face big challenges of inductive problem-solving. Policy options are ideally the creative result of a process of inductive problem-solving in which insights must be progressively and systematically built from elaboration of a large body of evidence. It is hard to generate insights into the policy challenges and the policy solutions unless the data from the different kinds of evidence are arranged in ways that are congenial to this inductive process. Putting evidence into boxes by way of orderly arrangement of paragraphs, sections, chapters, and parts of the report, can help the researcher make the connections critical to generating insights into solutions. Thus, the construction of a tightly hierarchical policy story involves a summarizing and re-summarizing of different kinds of evidence at different levels (paragraphs, sections, chapters, and parts) to encourage analytical commentary and inductive reasoning. A sound hierarchical structure may make it harder for researchers to fall into errors that are about not connecting evidence to findings and options.

Again, some of the most senior practitioners of the art of policy writing can be vulnerable to criticisms that there are faults in their inductive reasoning.

When this occurs, what went wrong? The 'vagueness' with which the Acheson report was charged was described this way:

> . . . some of the recommendations are simply too vague to be useful. Recommending "measures to prevent suicide among young people" or "policies to reduce the fear of crime and violence" would receive universal support but are of little use if it is not specified how these things are to be brought about. For example, the report advocates the development of a high quality affordable public transport system and specifically refers to the large relative increases in rail fares compared with motoring costs, but it fails to make the obvious link with the privatisation of the railways and the deteriorating service and increasing costs which have followed from the elementary logic that the creation of short term profits depends on emptying the purses of those who depend on, or chose, public transport.[249] (p. 1466)

This so-called 'vagueness' of recommendations is a problem that hierarchical ordering of evidence can help address by providing a means for induction of the evidence. This approach to ordering can help the researcher make not simply logical links between the large body of evidence in the report and the solutions, but also develop the *specificity* of the solutions induced. Thus, a tightly hierarchical policy story can help make findings more specific as the policy story is elaborated at different levels of the research report. It does not confer protection against politically motivated attacks on the quality of the research—but it can make such attacks more difficult to mount.

Being able to write the first draft of a policy-relevant report in a tight hierarchical structure takes time and an effort of application. It involves a particular approach to the composition of writing, which is often done at high speed in public sector policy units. The author has used the hierarchical model of meaning-making not to teach literacy, but rather to help highly literate people write for policy-makers in ways that meet policy-makers' expectations of highly organized hierarchical meaning-making.

Recommended reading

Stone D. *Policy Paradox: The Art of Political Decision-Making*. New York, W.W. Norton, 2002.

Case studies in policy story-telling

Case study: Making the policy argument for healthy ageing in the Netherlands

In the document *Policy for Older Persons in the Perspective of an Ageing Population*,[252] the government of the Netherlands deals with the challenge of a presenting policy for a sustainable 'whole-of-systems' approach to ageing in this country. It is less a research paper than a synthesis of research evidence to provide a policy argument for the government's approach to ageing.

The paper draws upon the results of existing international literature, as well as the results of studies conducted for the report into perceptions of ageing by the Dutch population, research into existing health and allied health services, as well as research into future scenarios such as housing needs relevant to the ageing Dutch population. The research involved on site visits and consultations with stakeholders and expert groups.

The policy argument made seeks to write back against a popular enabling assumption of health myths: that older people are less capable of participating in society. The report points out that this assumption is often present implicitly in the language in which old age is described:

> Both as this government's vision took shape and during the discussions with different partners, the view began to emerge that perhaps we are too inclined to see old age and population ageing as a problem, as a fate that will befall us: 'The problem of the labour participation rate of older people'; 'the problem of the costs of an ageing population for healthcare'; 'the problem of the social participation of older persons'; 'the problem of income for older people'; et cetera, et cetera. 'And population ageing will only increase the social consequences of the problem'. Viewed from this perspective, it does indeed seem that all senior citizens are no longer capable of working, are sick and lonely and have problems with their income. In essence, this view says that we do not expect much more from our senior citizens.[252] (p. 5)

The report also argues that it is in the common interests of Dutch society that older citizens be supported to participate fully in Dutch society. The inducements it offers in making this argument are that many benefits accrue to a society that works together to ensure this participation: increasing life expectancy, a healthier ageing population, increased workforce participation, increased standards of education of the ageing population, increased financial independence, home occupancy and other material independence of the ageing population. Thus, the report argues that supporting the participation of older citizens in Dutch society leads to an 'enrichment' of that society.

The report also offers other kinds of inducements in elaborating the practical aspects of its policy vision for ageing in the Netherlands. For example, in emphasising the value of supporting older citizens to stay fit and healthy, the report sets out a wide range of initiatives and incentives, including the extension of existing successful projects.

The policy argument in the report also makes use of rules and codes relevant to Dutch society. For example, it calls upon Dutch society's sense of fair play as well as its strong history of recognition of human rights in making the argument that it is unfair to appropriate and marginalize people simply because they are older:

> Our senior citizens are capable of very many things, and they want to do very many things. What is more, their valuable competencies and diversity make them a group that will not tolerate being universally labelled vulnerable and dependent.[252] (p. 5)

The report is also structured by a 'life-course' argument about ageing: that a pro-active approach to ageing in a society involves engaging with all the factors (such as investment in sustainable economic growth) necessary to achieve the well-being of an ageing population, now and for future generations of older citizens. By taking a futures perspective on ageing (not just addressing the needs of the current or immediate future ageing subpopulation), the report appeals to the interests of the whole community.

The report presents its argument weaving together a wide range of facts. For example, it pieces together facts about community opinion as well as demographic facts to create 'snapshots' of different historical moments in the history of the Netherlands: '1955: old in a country undergoing (re-) construction', '1980: old in a welfare state', '2005: old in an individualized society'.[252] (pp. 12–13) These help present the argument that the cultural and economic contexts of ageing have changed so much in the last 50 years that Dutch society needs a new approach to ageing.

Number sign systems are important to this report in the discursive text of the argument and in various charts. Numbers are often used whenever a certainty or a highly likely eventuality needs to be presented. For example, the report shows that, under different population scenarios, there will be increases in the numbers of ageing persons. This information is juxtaposed with information about social values and attitudes to highlight the need for change to approaches to ageing in the Netherlands: 'A shrinking workforce is being asked to generate the wealth to fund the provisions for a growing population of retirees. This imbalance is taking a heavy toll on the solidarity between the different generations.'[252] (p. 27) This discussion leads to the presentation of Dutch social values with reference to the European Constitution, including

> That 'older persons' who become vulnerable due to health problems, for example as a result of psycho-geriatric complaints, are assured of adequate and high-quality care provision, even if their numbers increase significantly due to population ageing. (p. 44)

In these and many other ways, the report uses language in a policy argument that could be described as populist, aiming to appeal to the sense of rights, shared values and responsibilities of the wider population. For example, it uses the first person plural 'our' to reinforce the idea that it presents the consensual views of Dutch society (the archetypal collective voice of the community) which has a shared stake in healthy ageing.[252] A critical aspect of this populist narrative technique is presenting research evidence in a way that invites the reader in the wider Dutch community to reflect on the nature of the challenges or 'rocks and hard places' that the society as a whole must face in reaching agreement that the approach the report outlines is the best possible one.

The report concludes with consideration of how the vision, including its operational details, might be communicated and implemented through particular mechanisms. This last part of the report describes how, for example, the Ministry of Health Welfare and Sport will work in collaboration with other ministries to create social debate and cohesion around the longer term aspects of the vision. As such it tries to offer a language in which policy-makers and the community can see how the policy vision can be realized and sustained.

Case study: Using language sign systems to educate—the case for a culture of patient safety in Ireland

The management of human error in the delivery of healthcare services is a key policy challenge facing many countries. In 2007, in the context of public concern about adverse events, the government of Ireland faced this challenge by establishing a commission that reported on reforms needed for patient safety and quality in the 2008 report *Building a Culture of Patient Safety*.[253]

The terms of reference of the commission required it to develop proposals for a system of governance that would include a framework for the implementation of managerial and clinical standards. The framework was to have legal, managerial, administrative, technical, and human resources measures.

At the heart of the argument being made in the report is the idea that it is possible to build a blame-free reporting and management culture and that a regard for patient safety can drive healthcare reform. This policy argument uses logic and rhetorical persuasion to build the legitimacy of its recommendations. It takes a strongly heuristic or educational approach to its reader, offering explanations and conceptualizations of patient safety and quality assurance with reference to a wide range of sources, national and international.

First, the report explores the background to the establishment of the commission. It argues that although failures in the Irish health system inform its work, it has taken a proactive approach based on international best practice and sound previous initiatives in the Irish healthcare system. The report adds legitimacy to its approach by detailing the results of its consultative process which involved a public call for submissions leading to identification of key issues that were of concern to the Irish community. The report then elaborates the nature of the patient safety and quality framework appropriate for Ireland. It identifies the values, such as patient centeredness and evidence-based practice, which should underpin the framework. It conceptualizes the elements of good governance.

The report then outlines how the Irish healthcare system might be made more participative for patients, carers and family members, including how the 'knowledgeable patient' might be developed. It explains what is open communication and why, despite obstacles such as a litigious patient culture, it might be better established in healthcare. The report explores what is the nature and purpose of leadership as part of effective governance and safety management, arguing for strong clinical leadership at the local and national levels. It models how reporting and accountability relationships should work (and be made explicit) for good governance, with vertical and horizontal integration, locally and nationally, outlining statutory relationships and responsibilities. However, pre-empting stakeholder concerns, it explains how a period of consultation will be needed before its proposed licensing framework is rolled out to diverse healthcare settings.

The report also argues for, and outlines, an integrated, lifelong, competencies-based approach to education, training, and research on patient safety, beginning at undergraduate level for health professionals. It examines how the current licensing system works in Ireland and available models for licensing (healthcare accreditation using agreed-upon standards) in other countries. It argues that while there is no evidence for a direct connection between licensing and healthcare quality, Ireland would be best served by a licensing system that takes a focus on continuous quality improvement processes. The report then examines professional regulation in Ireland and other countries, arguing for better separation of function as well as measures to correct gaps in the system. It also examines the operation of the system of professional recruitment, in Ireland and elsewhere, and identifies measures for tracking relevant information about a professional's performance.

The report also explains what is clinical effectiveness and how it might be achieved as part of an integrated quality assurance system. It explores what is an evidence-based approach to healthcare and what organizational arrangements might facilitate it. It elaborates the nature and role of clinical auditing, in Ireland and other countries, and makes suggestions for how clinical auditing capacities can be better established in Ireland. The report also examines the international evidence for error reporting, arguing for further development of the Irish system towards a mandatory reporting system for adverse events that is complemented by a voluntary reporting system for 'close calls' or 'near-misses'. It examines specific issues in medication safety, and how measures to manage and prevent medication error can be integrated into the Irish system in ways that build on existing initiatives. The report touches on the role of healthcare settings in patient safety and quality, and recommends further research. Finally, the report explains the role of information and information technology in creating the knowledgeable patient, highlighting ways in which the Irish system can be developed.

The report suggests that the Irish system faces significant reforms to achieve safety and quality, primarily through a more regulated system in line with agreed-upon national standards and policy objectives. It prioritizes legislative reforms led by an implementation steering committee with expert sub-groups.

The progress of this policy argument is hastened with typographical devices: strategic use of headings to summarize key arguments, italicized text to emphasize quotable quotes, shaded text boxes to highlight critical details, venn and flow diagrams to aid conceptualization, as well as tables to compare different quality assurance systems. As such it suggests an important dimension of policy writing that is not so well-emphasized in the policy literature—the use of language to conceptualize, educate, and 'make real' the steps needed to reform healthcare systems facing complex challenges such as safety and quality.

Case study: Weaving numbers and words to make an argument for hospital reform in the United Kingdom

The report *Hospital Guide 2008: The Health of our Hospitals Revealed* [254] was published by 'Dr Foster Intelligence' a public–private organization established in 2006 in the United Kingdom to improve public access to information about health and social care, most notably in the area of clinical performance, patient safety, quality, and mortality. The Hospital Guide 2008 is part of a series on hospital performance first published in 2001 with considerable media attention.

The primary data sources the report uses are the routine data submitted by the NHS (Commissioning Data Sets or CDS) and the annual questionnaire that Dr Foster Intelligence circulates to all English NHS trusts.

The data analyses used include the Hospital Standardized Mortality Ratio (HSMR). The report claims its usefulness lies in the identification of 'outliers' in both a positive or negative sense (though these are not done for trial indicators). Analyses are by different kinds of trusts (primary as well as acute).

The report focuses on three dimensions of quality that were meaningful in health policy at the time of its publication, notably in *High Quality Care for All: NHS Next Stage Review Final Report* [255]: patient safety, effectiveness of care, and patients' experiences (the NHS Next Stage Review also features as a case study in Chapter 9). For each of these, and with frequent reference to the change agenda emerging from the NHS Next Stage Review, the report presents selected indicators (both established as well as trial indicators) against which it analyses performance across the English NHS. Illumination of the policy problem and the meaning of findings also take place with reference to the key policy objectives of the Blair government, established clinical standards in the literature, and the history of international and UK developments and data trends in key areas of policy interest.

The report includes an upfront summary that makes the policy-relevant implications of the findings explicit. In this summary, the report synthesizes the data in accessible language and figures to identify where the NHS system is doing well and where it is not doing so well along the three dimensions of interest to policy decision-makers. For example, the report includes the following two observations under the dimension of 'effectiveness of care':

- ◆ focus on surgery for fractured neck of femur: there is wide variation in compliance with the standard that patients with a broken hip should have surgery within 2 days
- ◆ in four trusts, more than 80% of patients had surgery within 2 days. However, five trusts met this standard for no more than 30% of patients. (p. 7)

The main discussion in the report also includes the results of interviews with staff in the NHS, to allow triangulation and elaboration of the meaning of the quantitative data. It includes quotations from the CEOs of different NHS trusts offering contextual information helpful to understanding the significance of the performance data it presents. Performance data is also elaborated with the results of audits undertaken for case notes. This qualitative information is juxtaposed with graphs charting performance in particular areas (such as extraction of cataract activity over time in specific trusts). Non-shaded boxes offer quick 'grabs' of key performance data such as which trusts have the lowest rates of mastectomies. Shaded boxes are used to offer non-technical explanations of the graphs, and statistical debates about performance measures, as well as elaboration of other useful information to do with the study (such as analyses of the policy challenge presented by particular quality assurance reporting requirements, or descriptions of innovative approaches to quality assurance put in place by particular trusts). Layperson explanations of clinical procedures are offered in the text in ways that highlight the significance of performance data findings. Top performing trusts are also identified and showcased in the report, with photographs.

Throughout the report findings are presented in a manner that accounts for the question of how the data might properly be used in decision-making. For example, where variation in the data may be due to a range of factors not simply attributable to performance (such as poor coding of data) the report states:

We would recommend that trusts use these data analyses as a starting point to identify potential areas of concern and then use local audit techniques, such as the IHI's global trigger tool, to find out whether there really is a problem.[254] (p. 17)

It should be emphasized that doubts have been raised about some aspects of the validity and usefulness of these 'hospital mortality league tables'.[256] The report itself acknowledges gaps and challenges such as the lack of data from patients about their experiences of care.[254] However, it does offer a particularly pointed example of how to weave quantitative data into a policy story that speaks to policy decision-makers and the wider community.

Case study: Healthy People 2010 and using causality in policy arguments in the United States

The report *Healthy People 2010: Understanding and Improving Health*[257] may be used to explore some aspects of the art of policy story-telling. It is worth noting that the objectives set by earlier versions of this style of reporting *Healthy People 2000*[258] have been only partially achieved in the United States, which has actually seen declines in some areas of health.[259] *Healthy People 2010*[257] is essentially a statement of national health goals with specific objectives to be achieved by 2010. It was designed to be used as an instrument to improve health in the first decade of the new century, including at the level of local health planning and policy development. Essentially, the policy arguments being put relate to these policy goals.

First, using simple population health data, the report explores and justifies the view that not only are sound health outcomes important for Americans generally, but they also need to be achieved for particular equity target groups. The report begins by pointing out the importance to the American population of quality and years of healthy life, before considering related issues to do with health disparities. For example, it points out that there are at least 18 countries with populations of at least one million that have higher life expectancies than the United States.[257] The report also uses a simple line graph to make the argument that the lower the household income, the higher the likelihood that a person will self-report their health as fair or poor.[257] It presents key summary statistics using bar charts about disparities in health outcomes by health, race and ethnicity, income and education, disability, geographic location, and sexual orientation. This is part of an argument that 'every person in every community across the nation deserves equal access to comprehensive, culturally competent, community-based healthcare systems that are committed to serving the needs of the individual and promoting community health.'[257] (p. 16).

However, the report remains silent on the systemic influences on health outcomes. It models goals and related objectives as if local health policy and planning will be enough to overcome health disparities in the United States. It argues under a section beginning 'Determinants of health' that 'individual and environmental factors are responsible for about 70% of all premature deaths in the United States'[257] (p. 18). It lists the determinants of health as 'biology', 'behaviours', 'social environment', 'physical environment', 'policies and interventions', and 'access to quality healthcare' without discussing the systemic economic determinants of health. This paves the way for the implicit policy argument that reaching the health goals in 2010 is all about acting to remove these barriers to good health. Thus, the report argues that 'understanding and monitoring behaviours, environmental factors, and community health systems may prove more useful to monitoring the Nation's true health, and in driving health improvement activities'[257] (p. 21). But income is considered more as a function of individual circumstances than as the outcome of systemic economic forces acting on the individual. The role of the health indicators in the report is to act as a framework for policy and to 'motivate action' albeit of a particular kind[257] (p. 24). For example, one of the objectives listed for the indicator 'Access to healthcare' is 'Increase the proportion of persons with health insurance'[257] (p. 44). The discussion supporting this objective points out that 'More than 44 million persons in the United States do not have health insurance, including 11 million uninsured children'. It states that a financial barrier is 'not having health insurance' and a structural barrier is 'lack of healthcare facilities' but remains silent on systemic market forces that act to reduce access of the poor to health services[257] (p. 45). Thus, the report is essentially a policy argument for a particular view of the causes of health disparities which excludes wider systemic economic forces acting to prevent affordable healthcare cover for many Americans.

Chapter 8

Writing sound health policy options

Overview

This chapter offers ideas for delivering policy options that are designed to meet decision-makers' needs. The chapter offers conceptual understandings of what are policy options and uses exemplars from research reports for policy-makers to analyse the different forms that policy options can take.

The challenge of delivering health policy options

While there are many research publications on policy analysis, it is difficult to find a single paper or book on the art of actually writing policy options. Policy options can be defined as the concise summary of decisions that need to be made by policy decision-makers, which are most strongly supported by the relevant considerations: not just research evidence, both formal and informal, but also political and strategic considerations.

Writing options for health policy is not the same as writing broad 'conclusions' and 'directions for future research' that belong in genres of scholarly writing. In scholarly genres conclusions about the policy actions that need to be taken are often at best an after thought, 'tacked on' to the research evidence. Leading UK policy researchers conclude that the traditional form of research recommendations is possibly of limited value for policy-makers because a whole range of factors beyond empirical evidence must be weighed into such conclusions-finding.[81] Rarely does the writing of conclusions for scholarly papers involve social practices of auditing options for policy-making through knowledge brokering and negotiation with stakeholders, and weighing diverse considerations from legal regulations to community values to model useful solutions.

Key ideas

Policy-makers are interested in highly creative and innovative policy options that emerge from diverse forms of evidence, weighed for their strengths and weakness as solutions to particular policy challenges in particular contexts. The challenge in research for policy is to present policy options that are evidence-driven, but allow policy-makers scope to exercise values and their own political judgments in changing contexts.

In policy-relevant research, developing the policy options can place the heaviest impost on the researcher's creative, strategic, conceptual, people, and problem-solving skills.

Models for understanding what is a policy decision

The nature of what happens when a policy-maker makes a policy decision is poorly understood. Yet it is known that this form of decision-making can be very complex. It is not a matter of simply 'adding up' the empirical evidence. As Steven Lewis has observed, 'Evidence often makes decision-making more difficult, not less' because 'Where the outcome distributions overlap, there is a zone of uncertainty'. He concludes that 'Decisions and frameworks to guide them are the product of deliberation, not ratiocination'[110] (p. 168).

Bearing in mind the discussion of incremental models for policy-making noted in Chapter 1, the work of Majone offers a basis for conceptualizing a policy decision as a core set of unchangeable conditions as well as a range of adaptable elements:

> What gives a policy stability is that some of its values, assumptions, methods, goals, and programmes are held to be central and only to be abandoned, if at all, under the greatest stress and at the risk of severe internal crises. What gives the policy adaptability is that many values, assumptions, methods, goals, and programmes are disposable, modifiable, or replaceable by new ones.[16] (p. 150)

At the same time, the core aspects of the policy context may be in a state of progressive dismantling at the periphery.

Key ideas

Majone's conceptualization of core and peripheral or changeable elements offers a model of policy decision-making that is essentially about making an informed decision about what is core and what is peripheral at a particular time.[16] It is as much about deciding what to change as what not to.

Clearly though, a policy decision includes a powerful element of deciding what might work under what kind of changed conditions. In a realist review perspective (as described in Chapter 3) policy options are conceptualized not as delivering up a synthesis of 'what works' but rather of modelling decision paths that might be taken under particular conditions.[84]

The work of Charles Ragin described in Chapter 5 offers a basis for reflecting on the combinatorial nature of policy decision-making.[161] For example, policy-makers often want to draw lessons from diverse models that work in different ways in different contexts. The question they are often asking is 'Which elements of what health models will work to meet this particular combination of policy challenges with what results for my local context?' Thus the policy options should deliver solutions in a form that answers this question, as suggested by the discussion later in this chapter.

The content of policy options

The content of policy options can be conceptualized as including content to do with persuasion and explanation. The persuasive content is about justifying a particular policy option. The explanatory content is about implementation of the policy options. The policy options can be positive or negative i.e. they can be about undertaking a course of action or not undertaking or prohibiting certain courses of action as part of maintaining core areas of policy, as Majone has noted.[16]

The persuasive content can suggest the strengths and weakness of each policy option. It can be conceptualized as an effort to substantiate or justify the policy options by comparing summaries of these strengths and weaknesses. In line with the discussion on structuring the research report given in the last chapter, it is often critical that such summaries emerge logically from the body of the report. They should include the whole raft of relevant considerations. The researcher will need to decide how much and what kinds of information to present, for example, about the economic costs of the policy options. Such details can be given in an appendix or the body of the report in a dedicated section, and given in essence in the summaries for the policy options.

The content of policy options can also include information about uncertainty. The variability of policy contexts means that the policy option will almost inevitably be a decision taken in a context of uncertainty. The challenge of uncertainty was discussed in Chapter 2 on deciphering the policy problem. The content of policy options can include supporting information about not only what is known, but also what, at the end of the research process, is unknown or uncertain about each of the policy options (both positive and negative). Such information can have persuasive power for policy-makers who are willing to embrace greater or lesser degrees of risk in the light of other information about strengths and weaknesses of a particular policy option.

Summary information about the sustainability of each policy option can also have powerful persuasive value. As Chapter 4 suggested, when weighing the value of a particular policy option, health policy-makers are often also concerned with the question of whether the option being proposed is sustainable. Such information ideally is collected as part of review, data collection, and analysis exercises. If this is done, the policy solutions can also summarize relative information on the sustainability of each option.

The explanatory content about implementation of policy solutions can suggest who will do what, when, how. This does not mean that all the thinking through of implementation needs to be done. It does mean that the solutions need to include summary information linked to more extensive evidence in the body of the report.

For example, information about timelines can be an important part of this kind of explanatory modelling of policy options. As has been noted elsewhere in this book, policy options do have a 'shelf-life' and the typical election cycle is likely to influence policy-makers. This does not mean options with longer-term implementation timelines cannot be included. It does mean that including longer-term policy options often places an impost on researchers to link those options to succinct summaries of evidence in the report about their return for policy-makers (not just specific interest groups). This evidence can include hard information about broader inter-sectoral community support and demonstrable sustainability.

Key practical strategies

Thus, the content of options can be designed to include summaries of strengths and weakness of each option, including information about uncertainty and sustainability, as well as information about implementation and timelines.

The form of policy solutions: options and recommendations

I'm more comfortable with broad ranges of type of approach than just definitive answers . . . if you get to a single answer then your ability to interpret that within your system is much more difficult. Of course, the flip side to that is, that's where part of the problem emerges because you get broad bandings for policy and people interpret

> broad bandings within the environment they are in, so you continue to get variation
> in the way policy emerges and is developed.
>
> (health agency CEO)

The discussion so far has used the term 'policy options'. However, care should be taken to distinguish policy options from recommendations. They both summarize the policy decisions that can be taken—the policy solutions. In practice, the two forms can overlap. However, recommendations and options can be quite different depending on the degrees of complexity of the policy solutions being represented. Recommendations are shorter, more singular, one dimensional statements of what policy decisions need to be taken. Policy options tend to be longer, made up of different parts and multi-dimensional. They can often include summary tabs. A summary tab is a short descriptive sentence distilling the information in the body of the report. Summary tabs can be presented in tables under different headings for each policy option.

Deciding the form of policy solutions

Again, uncertainty plays an important role in deciding the form of the policy solutions. Identifying what that uncertainty is and providing for it is part of designing policy solutions. The map of the nature of uncertainty outlined in Chapter 2 with the suggestion that the researcher use it throughout the research can be updated, using the research findings, and used for the purposes of designing the policy solutions.

Very uncertain high stakes policy contexts may need policy solutions modelled as flexible decisions that are robust enough to work across different situations i.e. policy options. Policy options can take the form of core elements and supplementary elements that can be combined in different ways. This flexibility can assist policy-makers to make the necessary trade-offs between different kinds of information about what is known and unknown.

However, some policy contexts may require more one-dimensional policy options styled as recommendations, as for example, when the researcher has been directed to deliver singular solutions or when all the relevant considerations point in a single direction. In practice though, most policy-making contexts will have sufficient complexity and uncertainty to suggest the value of using the combinatorial form of policy options.

Designing combinatorial policy options

The combinatorial form of policy options can involve three to five policy options, each of which can have core elements as well as supplementary elements. Each policy option can offer a different combination of these elements.

In this approach, the researcher would first identify the set of core and supplementary elements needed for designing the different policy options.

The core elements are often developed from areas where the evidence is strongest: areas of community consensus, areas where local and international experience including strategic and political considerations are most favourable. Using Majone's conceptualization of policy decision-making, the core elements can also be associated with aspects of a policy context that are held to be central and provide for continuity of a system.[16]

The supplementary elements are often useful to making trade-offs between different kinds of considerations. Again, using Majone's conceptualization of policy-making, the supplementary elements may also be associated with aspects of policy context that are modifiable and replaceable.[16]

Key practical strategy

A viable combinatorial policy option is one that offers both core and supplementary elements, so that policy-makers can clearly see possibilities for trade-offs in ways that do not jeopardize the elements that are critical to the success of policy options and central to the viability of a policy context.

Negotiating for support for, and testing, the policy solutions

The literature emphasizes the value of testing policy options and recommendations with key stakeholders. Chapter 6 on consensus-building for health policy offered many practical strategies and techniques for working with stakeholders to develop consensus around the policy solutions. That chapter can be used to develop strategies for auditing and testing emerging options with health stakeholders, as well as knowledge brokering to gain support for preferred options.

Recommended reading

Majone G. *Evidence, Argument & Persuasion in the Policy Process*. USA, Yale University Press, 1989.

Case studies in designing policy solutions

Case study: Combating Methamphetamine in the state of Minnesota—broad recommendations for action

Methamphetamine has a major impact on many communities, including in the state of Minnesota, United States. The 2008 report *Methamphetamine in Minnesota: A Report on the Impact of One Illicit Drug*[260] provided an evaluation of the impact, costs, initiatives and progress made in this area in Minnesota. Its policy solutions were delivered in the form of broad one line recommendations, with accompanying paragraphs offering further elaboration of the nature of, and need for, each individual recommendation.

For example, recommendation 8 was: 'Clarify substance abuse data restrictions and provide training'[260] (p. 48). The elaboration offered was as follows:

> At virtually every cross-disciplinary meeting of professionals involved with substance abuse prevention, enforcement, and treatment, concerns are expressed about the restrictions imposed by government data practices laws regarding what data may be shared and what must be kept private. There seems to be a widespread belief that these restrictions seriously inhibit overall substance abuse efforts. This is particularly critical in connection with rescuing and protecting drug-endangered children. In some cases, there is a lack of information or lack of clarity about the data practices laws, not necessarily an actual prohibitive restriction. A comprehensive effort to provide information and training on data practices to the various professionals who work on substance abuse issues would help maximize the effectiveness of substance abuse resources and help protect those endangered by drug abuse.[260] (p. 48)

This form of recommendation may be helpful when a single issue such as methamphetamine needs to be engaged with across a broad range of areas. It may also be appropriate for developing a broad framework for action, prior to consideration of the detail of implementation.

Case study: More detailed policy solutions for developing the quality and safety of maternity services in New Zealand

Following a sentinel event (the death of a baby), the Director-General of Health in New Zealand commissioned an independent review, reported in *A Review of the Quality, Safety and Management of Maternity Services in the Wellington Region*. The review offers detailed policy solutions engaging with systemic issues in the Wellington region, however, it also offers implications for the development of maternity services nationally.[261]

The review was overseen by a four-person, clinician-led expert team that aimed to examine the adequacy (quality and safety) of maternity services in the Wellington region and identify any opportunities for improvement. The scope of the review included accountability arrangements, as well as systems and procedures applying to maternity providers. The review methodology was primarily qualitative: document reviews, interviews with stakeholders, observation and site visits, as well as a review of over 140 community submissions.[261]

The report offered different kinds of findings and policy solutions for the attention of policy-makers. First, it provided broad conclusions in the form of 13 bullet points that directly addressed the issue of the safety and quality of maternity services in the Wellington area: for example, that 'maternity services in the Wellington area are as safe as maternity services anywhere else in New Zealand' and 'Some components of an effective quality management system are in place but the management of quality and risk needs to be significantly improved.'[261] (p. 8)

Second, the report provided seven bullet points that offered broad implications of the review for maternity services more generally for New Zealand: for example, that 'To ensure safety for women and their babies, and appropriate support for new graduate midwives, there needs to be mandatory supervision (physical oversight) and mentoring for midwives in their first year of practice.'[261] (p. 9)

Third, the report also provided a tabled list of commendations of aspects of both the regional Wellington and the national New Zealand maternity services systems, so that policy-makers could be informed about what was working well. For example, the report advised that 'Wellington Hospital Delivery Suite provides Kenepuru with very good (immediate) access to specialist obstetric advice by telephone when this is required' and 'The Midwifery Council of New Zealand and the New Zealand Colleague of Midwives are commended for implementing robust competence requirements and review processes for midwives.'[261] (p. 9)

Fourth, the report provided a table with 18 detailed policy solutions relating to maternity services in the Wellington area. Each of these was given a descriptor, a risk rating, a nominated agency for implementation, and a timeline. For example, the report advised 'That the midwifery leader be present at management meetings on an equal footing with the clinical director Women's and Child Health, and contribute equally to decision-making about maternity services'; this was given a 'moderate' risk rating as an action to be implemented by the Capital and Coast District Health Board by October 2008 (the same month the report was published).

Finally, the report provided a table with 19 policy solutions relating to national issues for New Zealand maternity services. These were similar in structure to the recommendations for the Wellington area. However, the descriptors were often longer than a sentence, offering a summary of the issue and then one or more preferred solutions.

The policy solutions provided in the report were not designed to present alternative judgements but rather the complement and extend one another as part of a 'whole-of-system' approach to improving New Zealand's regional and national maternity system. As such they offered an integrated approach that nonetheless gave policy-makers some flexibility.

Case study: Promoting Health in Hong Kong—a detailed strategic framework for action on non-communicable diseases

The increase in the number of people suffering from non communicable diseases (NCDs) such as diabetes, heart disease, and cancer, presents a major health policy challenge to do with the complexities of lifestyle and behaviour change. The report *Promoting Health in Hong Kong: A Strategic Framework for Prevention and Control of Non-communicable Diseases* suggests one way in which policy solutions can be conceptualized and presented as part of a government-led community discussion of directions for action in tackling a complex health challenge.

The report presented a 'Non-Communicable Diseases Prevention and Control Strategic Framework' that synthesizes the work of government researchers and over 40 experts across different sectors and disciplines. The research base for the report is comprised of a conceptual discussion as well as an analysis of 'what works', drawing on the international literature, as well as discussion of overseas models and recommendations of the World Health Organization. Data profiling the Hong Kong population and related health promotion and disease activities are also included.[262]

The strategic framework itself focuses on major preventable or modifiable risk factors as part of an 'upstream' approach. It is informed by a vision of a well-informed population, a caring community, competent healthcare professionals, and a sustainable healthcare system. The framework sets out some clear goals to do with, for example, creating an environment conducive to promoting health, and reducing avoidable hospital admissions and healthcare procedures.[262]

The strategic framework offers six broad strategic directions. For example, 'direction 1' is 'Support new and strengthen existing health promotion and NCD prevention initiatives or activities that are in line with this strategy'. 'Direction 6' is 'Strengthen and develop supportive health promoting legislation'.[262] (p. xii) Each of the strategic directions is supported by a set of actions: for example, 'direction 1' is supported by an action 'fostering implementation of territory-wide health promotion programmes such as 'healthy eating', 'active living' and 'tackling overweight'".[262] (p. 63) The key elements for implementation are conceptualized in terms of community partnerships, a whole-of-environment approach, health outcomes, population-based interventions, a whole-of-life approach, and empowerment. The report provides illustrative case studies and explanations in boxes under these concepts. The report also contains information about how to implement the framework through a strategic management infrastructure comprised of a steering group and working groups, detailing specific objectives and tasks.[262]

Thus the report presents a 'package' approach to policy solutions: a tightly integrated whole-of-systems set of actions, in ways that aim to help policy-makers conceptualize and see how to achieve the policy solutions being proposed.

Chapter 9

Maximizing the dissemination and impact of evidence for health policy

Overview

Chapter 1 gave an overview of some models of research transfer in the policy literature. This final chapter takes up that discussion again, exploring how researchers can understand and use the policy change process to actively manage the dissemination and impact of their research.

The elements of dissemination

. . . you go through all this work and then that research sits on our shelf . . . if it's solid research then it does need to be revisited. But you know with our society and the time constraints and the information overload that already exists, I don't know how you do that. I've watched our Health Care Commission which has done a lot of research on various projects here, and we have spent a lot of money. I can think of one study that we did, three or four years ago. I don't think it was a bad piece of work, but for a lot of reasons that six hundred thousand or nine hundred thousand dollars of research will never be looked at again. Part of it is it gets outdated very quickly. Part of it is people and policy makers change because of the election cycles and because of job turnover. And pretty soon nobody even remembers that that research was done, let alone possibly pulling it off the shelf as a resource so that that sort of research doesn't get a chance to be looked at again . . . that's very frustrating.

(health agency CEO)

University research assessment systems in many countries tend to encourage researchers to build expertise in getting published in peer-reviewed international journals. They tend not to encourage researchers to build expertise in disseminating their research findings for the purposes of policy-making.[33] However, successful policy-relevant research also involves translating findings into different forums to maximize the influence of research. The importance of this aspect of research for policy cannot be over-stated. In the United Kingdom, for example, many government departments require research submissions to ministers and senior public servants to include explanation of how the policy being advocated will be communicated to the community.[144] The applied policy literature in particular suggests that the marketing of policies may be an increasing feature of the 21st Century policy landscape. Policy design now includes policy marketing as an important part of providing for the complexities of dissemination.[144]

This chapter cannot hope to offer more than an outline of some key concepts and strategies for increasing the use of research. Readers are encouraged to consult the definitive book on the subject by Nutley, Walter, and Davies, *Using Evidence: How Research can Inform Public Services*.[36] This chapter emphases not just the dissemination of the written report in various media, but also the use of different social practices and relationship-building to maximize the take-up and impact of the research evidence. Thus, with reference to literature across the disciplines, as well as practical examples, this chapter offers theoretical and practical understandings of dissemination understood also as a strategic communication and social skill set. This social art includes knowledge brokering, finding and building local champions, building partnerships, shaping organizational cultures—all of which are important for maximizing the impact of research evidence and marketing the policies being advocated.

Key ideas

The strategic communication and social skill set important to the dissemination of research can be critical to its success. This success is measured by the extent to which a diverse community—often only initially policy decision-makers—respond to, and ideally champion and use, its policy options and recommendations. Managing the dissemination and impact of policy-relevant research can be very demanding, given that such research is by definition often about sensitive and controversial issues to do with systems change.

This chapter suggests that meeting that challenge is a task ideally done using a well-developed formal plan, as suggested by the 'translational science' model of research-practice-policy transfer. However, as Nutley, Walter, and Davies have suggested, the use of research is influenced by many other factors that can upset the best of well-laid plans.[36]

Dissemination defined

'Dissemination' is a complex concept that is only beginning to be defined. It is not well-defined for health policy-making purposes, which does present with related but different challenges of evidence dissemination. Certainly, the concept of dissemination does not just mean getting research 'known' in a public domain since that in itself is not sufficient to change policy. Dissemination also involves the utilization of research. That is, for dissemination of research to occur, there must be some kind of reaction or impact or implementation of the research.[263]

As Chapter 1 suggested, research can be said to be used in different senses: for example, when there is instrumental take-up, or when there is conceptual reworking of the policy-maker's understanding of the problem, or when there is political use to support a predetermined decision.[8] However, research use can also be conceptualized as a process of engagement between the researcher and communities of action (those who will decide and implement the policy) involving receiving, processing the research and applying the research findings.[264]

There are different kinds of applied models for maximizing research-policy transfer. These include the work done by centres for the dissemination of research and policy observatories, which give summaries of research in an accessible format. However, dissemination needs to be better theorized so that the assumptions upon which it is based can be questioned.

Theoretical frameworks for the dissemination of research into healthcare decision-making generally (i.e. for both policy and practice) suggest that it is influenced by individual, organizational, and environmental factors, as well as factors to do with the characteristics of the innovation itself.[265] These factors interact in complex ways as research evidence is disseminated in stages to do with knowledge about the innovation, persuasion, decision-making, implementation, and confirmation.[265] For example, the characteristics of the innovation may be that it is technical, or that it is more administrative: this will affect the rate at which it will be adopted, depending on the other interacting factors.[265] Such views of dissemination of research are drawn from Roger's Diffusion Theory suggesting that dissemination is a process occurring over time and comprised of a sequence of actions.[265, 266]

However, not all research can be considered an innovation. Not only that, but the process of dissemination may be more multi-dimensional or nonlinear than such models can readily convey.[36, 265] Accordingly, the main value of such models is to alert researchers to potential challenges and strategic issues in evidence dissemination. For example, organizational factors to do with the dissemination of the innovation being proposed by the research should be considered: factors to do with numbers and nature of staff, nature and extent of services, organizational location and culture, communication channels and decision-making processes, as well as other structural features of the organization may need to be considered.[265] The importance of considering how organizations work internally and together to shape what happens to research is also emphasized by Nutley, Walter, and Davies.[36]

The ways in which information can be used, and that use conceptualized, and the ways in which dissemination can be said to occur, are as varied as the information itself.

Key practical strategy

The work of Nutley, Walter, and Davies suggest that much theory on research use may fail to engage with the complexity of the process. They suggest that the circulation of findings from research to policy-makers and practitioners is only one of a range of strategies for helping to make sure that research is used. Other strategies include interaction (ongoing contact between researchers and policy-makers, knowledge brokering, negotiation, and dissemination of the research through direct ongoing dialogue); the use of influential figures to transmit the research; and facilitation (creating a context or media to facilitate research uptake). They also emphasize that dissemination of research does not happen at the end of the research production stage, but can be conceptualized as an ongoing part of the research,[36] as this book has emphasized. Above all, Nutley, Walter, and Davies remind researchers that an attention to the complexities of the context in which research is to be used—rather than a reliance on any one theory of how research is used—is the basis for a sound approach to maximizing its use.[36]

In this book, the aim of dissemination is to ensure that the policy options are actually accepted. They may not all be accepted, and they may be changed in the process, and/or they may be incrementally implemented, but if the research has quality and equity, the aim can be to ensure that they are substantively accepted.

Communities of action: a key challenge of dissemination

By now readers may agree that it is an obvious point to say that policy-makers, practitioners, and other community stakeholders ought to be involved in the production of the research, including research design, at the earliest stages if the research is to be disseminated properly. However, not least because this is not a straightforward matter, it is worth pointing out how this key assertion of this book is also important to a number of writings on knowledge dissemination.

'Knowledge Diffusion and Utilization' (KDU) theory and practice emphasizes the early involvement of those who are the potential knowledge users—not just in dissemination, but ideally in the conceptualization and conduct of the research.[267] By some accounts this involvement of users (decision-makers and implementers) in the design of research is the best means of achieving research dissemination and take-up at the end of the process.[267] The aim is to, by the end of the research process, have built a partnership of trust, ownership, and consensus.[267] It can be described as a kind of participative research for better dissemination. This insight is also central to the monograph on research use produced by Nutley, Walter, and Davies *Using Evidence: How Research can Inform Public Services.*[36] In their explanations of realist approaches to research for policy-making, Pawson and colleagues also emphasize the value of the researcher working with policy-makers and practitioners to develop policy options for particular contexts.[84] Accordingly, as this book has also emphasized, the process for creating knowledge must also include a participative process for ensuring the knowledge gets used.

However, there is some interesting evidence that when researchers interact with public health units to produce the research report, they increase knowledge of their research but not necessarily utilization of research. There may be greater understanding (receiving, reading, and information processing) when research users are involved in the production of research, and there may be an intention formed to use the research, but that does not mean that the research will actually be applied to effect a change.[264]

Key practical strategy

As the definition of dissemination just given suggested, for dissemination to occur, something more than involvement in aspects of the research or passive dissemination must happen. This 'something more' requires the researcher to engage in a kind of proactive, strategic dissemination to overcome obstacles to the research being implemented. Thus, the key challenge of dissemination is about making an iterative *strategic* process happen between the researcher and the communities of action, over time. This challenge will often involve engaging with the nature of the organizational climates in which the research will be disseminated, and any political and cultural issues. It also requires a commitment of resources.[263]

Developing the plan for dissemination

As noted in Chapter 4 on research methods, the development of a systematic plan for research-policy transfer is ideally a critical part of policy-relevant research. Studies of dissemination suggest that planning for dissemination should be done at the earliest stages of the research.[263] The assumption that research-policy-practice transfer requires strategic planning (rather than re-inventing methods) works well in policy contexts if the research that is to be translated is from the outset oriented to policy-maker's needs.

The dissemination plan should include practical initiatives for maximizing research transfer. The initiatives can be designed to help ensure that the dissemination will take place at all the levels that matter: at the local community and practice level, as well as at the systemic political and policy-making level, to keep the research current. Dissemination plans can also offer strategies for achieving dissemination by targeting: the source (knowledge-makers); the message (what is being said); the medium (how it is being said); the users of the research (policy-makers and community members).[263]

Key practical strategy

For example, in relation to

- the source: the dissemination of the research can be greatly aided by strategic choice of steering group members who can then act as conduits back to their respective communities

- the message: dissemination of research can be assisted by many of the substantive issues of research method for policy-making contexts explored in this book to address the policy problem

- the medium: dissemination can be facilitated by systematic mapping of the different genres and formats in which the evidence can be elaborated for different audiences: electronic discussion lists, feedback to study participants, interactive CD, internet, seminars and workshops, public meetings, presentations to professional groups, newsletters by email, posters, educational materials, and so on

- targeting users: dissemination can be facilitated by the participative research methods outlined in Chapter 6 as well as a range of systematically planned events such as launches of the report and use of personal and organizational incentives (of course, within ethical guidelines).

Each of these levels of, and ways of targeting, dissemination are complex and present challenges that ought not to be underestimated.

There are other ways of conceptualizing the dissemination plan. Knott and Wildavsky describe three broad action-based approaches to dissemination:

1 Moving information, so that it is more accessible to those with whom the researcher wants to communicate, for example, by establishing new kinds of information exchanges.

2 Moving people, by creating opportunities for people to interact in ways that are helpful to disseminating the research evidence.

3 Stimulating natural dissemination by developing incentives that help overcome the obstacles to diffusion of research evidence.[35]

Stakeholder and policy-makers should be closely involved in development of the dissemination plan itself. The plan should also be costed at the outset of the research.

The legal, regulatory, and protocol considerations that operate in a particular context need to be considered as part of the framework for dissemination of policy-relevant research. They should be figured into the plan for dissemination.

Using networks to disseminate research

Case studies of health research suggest the importance of social and policy networks not just to the conduct of research, but also its dissemination.[32] These networks can offer a way of understanding and harnessing the involvement of communities of action in the task of dissemination. Chapter 3 on reviewing the evidence outlined the nature of policy networks, a discussion that was picked up again in Chapter 4 on research methods and Chapter 6 on community consensus-building. The different kinds of networks discussed and methods for engaging with them can help the researcher design a process of dissemination—including overcoming obstacles to dissemination.

Studies of the dissemination of research among health professionals suggest that researchers need to have nuanced contextual information about how they work, in what ways, and for which professionals. Assumptions that these networks operate in similar ways are likely to be flawed.[263] For example, not only do doctor networks differ from nursing networks,[263, 268] but a single kind of network may show great variation. Some networks are highly centralized in the sense that they operate in hierarchies. Others are more decentralized with a number of major actors.[268] Such networks can include 'issue networks' of government insiders, academics, think tank policy experts, and media writers who act as knowledge brokers to different communities.[130] As Nutley, Walter, and Davies point out, there are 'intermediary broker organizations' that can help disseminate research and these can be critical to the task of dissemination. For example, organizations representing medical professionals can offer a conduit to not just practitioners, but also senior policy-makers. There are also various knowledge brokering organizations that may have been established by government, as well as think tanks and charitable agencies.[36]

At the outset of the research (not just at the end stage), the nature of key networks should be mapped with an awareness that such networks can be expected to be different for different occupational groups.[268] As Chapter 4 suggested, network theory and practice in political science and other disciplines is sufficiently advanced that networks for disseminating a particular policy innovation can be modelled using data-driven methods.[130] Internal networks (e.g. internal organizational networks) and external networks (such as regional, national, and international networks) can be identified in ways that allow consideration of, and sound choices about, how these different networks may affect the consideration and adoption of different policies.[130] Approaches to mapping such networks can be qualitative or quantitative, or both.

Key practical strategy

A useful model for identifying and studying networks is suggested by the UK-based work of West et al. who randomly surveyed members of health practice networks and asked respondents to name individuals with whom they had discussed important professional (clinical and managerial) matters.[268]

Such research can identify individuals who would be good targets for particular events aimed at co-opting the support of networks for the dissemination of the research in relatively small areas. Densely connected networks may present stronger supports for, or obstacles to, policy change.[268] Less densely connected networks may be useful to spreading information over longer distances but it may be wrong to assume they will be able to mobilize a particular group for a policy option without more resources being invested in that effort. Research into the functioning of policy networks can also identify particular cliques that may be relatively isolated, and thus may require more intensive approaches aimed at penetrating the group's boundaries.[268]

Forums for policy dissemination

. . . you have to throw a lot of spaghetti at the wall and then see what sticks, so it's email, it's trying to get a little article in the press, it's getting on public radio, it's doing briefings of key policy-makers, it's having a short two page summary, easy access to the longer report. I think—at least in my experience—the research entities that put a lot of marketing effort into their dissemination of their work are the ones that really have an impact on policy . . . we do a lot of little ninety minute briefings on topics where maybe three or four research briefs are presented and the actual researchers are there and people can ask them questions.

(health agency CEO)

Dissemination is also about the art of delivering evidence in different genres for different forums. Researchers can add value to research by including supplementary briefing papers for different audiences—from parliamentarians, to practitioners and community stakeholders, to the media. These will need to be carefully tailor-made to reflect the issues and language that is meaningful for these different groups:

. . . if a two hundred and fifty page book lands on my desk . . . it is quite difficult for me in a hospital environment to really take the learning from that. That might be a problem with our system or a problem with the way I work or whatever, but that's kind of the reality of it . . . it's the packaging of the results . . . that's one of the issues that has hampered research into practice.

(health agency CEO)

A critical element of dissemination planning is the media campaign, especially where there may be a need to put pressure on policy decision-makers. The work of Nelson, Hess, and Croyle offers a basis for understanding how to communicate health research to the media, especially quantitative research.[73] Researchers should consider also how to use the media to consensus-build: to find the 'angle' in often complex policy issues that can help the researcher use media releases and stories to create productive consensus around the preferred policy option. Much of the discussion on making policy arguments in Chapter 7 is relevant to this task.

Key practical strategy

Thus the plan for dissemination of the research should also include a plan for this kind of 'media advocacy' work: a plan for generating news media coverage of a particular issue in order to advocate a particular policy solution. Typically this is done as part of a broader approach to advocacy that includes networking, lobbying, community meetings, and so on.[269] Different models of media advocacy should be considered, depending on the nature of the policy outcome being sought.

Media advocacy can be undertaken by many different interests, however, it can also be undertaken by researchers. The fate of too many researchers in the media suggests how easily their well-intentioned messages about research can produce results that are damaging for them professionally and their work. Researchers and policy advisors in public sector research units often develop and sustain important relationships with local newspapers and television reporters that can help prevent this kind of problem. If the reporter who seeks the material is unknown to the researcher, it may be helpful to make submission of the final proposed news item to the researcher a condition of participation.

The work of implementation

This book has emphasized that the considerations of policy delivery must be a key part of policy design from its first inception.[18] Thus the work of implementation, or at least its design, needs to begin at the earliest stage of the design of the research for appraising the policy options. This is because the research evidence often needs to include comparative information about the viability of options, the manageability of risk and the extent to which benefits can be realized in practice.[72] Research reports for policy may not get implemented, or get improperly implemented, if the report does not offer the necessary cues on how to ensure its preferred options or recommendations are operationalized.

Key practical strategy

Some contexts may require the development of a detailed implementation plan for a particular policy option or options. This can include a timetable for delivering the policy including a 'sunset clause' when the policy must be reviewed or terminated, an outline of the roles and responsibilities of those who may need to be involved in delivering the policy (including guidelines for the implementation committee), money, skills, and infrastructure needed, strategies for overcoming particular barriers to implementation (including risks and uncertainties), as well as arrangements for reporting and monitoring performance.[144]

Researchers may be involved at some level in the implementation of the policy options. At the very least, they may have an information-giving and translation role, if they are called upon to explain different aspects of the report. Or they may have a quality assurance, monitoring, and evaluation role (though this is ideally done by researchers other than those who designed the policy options).

... where do you cut off? You might say 'Okay, we've had eighteen months, two years of this program, it's time now to cut the cord. It's not going to deliver. Nothing ventured, nothing gained. But time to dis-invest.' We're not good at that.

(health agency CEO)

The plan for dissemination of the research needs to include this evaluation element; too many policies are not sustained because there is not enough information about how well they have worked. The cycle of testing the success of a policy decision and refining and developing the implementation of that decision in the light of high quality advice is critical. Too many policies have also not been terminated or implemented improperly because this was not done.[144] The evaluation of a policy option can begin with a pilot or trial phase, with provision for stakeholder-driven feedback. Including a pilot or trial phase can also be helpful to assessing the likely costs of an option, as long as there is sufficient flexibility to modify the policy option in the light of such information.[144]

Translating policy research into scholarly research forums

Researchers might also like to give some thought to how to translate the policy-relevant research report into international scholarly publications. Too many community-based researchers struggle to acquire skills in translating their research into scholarly forums: they accumulate many project reports and little international scholarly recognition of their research. Some university-based researchers are also concerned that if they embark on community-based project work they will be hindered rather than helped to build an international profile of scholarly publications. This can be unhelpful to attracting quality researchers into applied policy research. Chapters 3 to 6 offered suggestions for how to design research that meets quality standards. Rigorous policy-relevant research has a far better chance of being translated into high quality international journals than poorly designed, context-bound research. As this book has aimed to convey, if research and policy exist in two different worlds they can at least meet in a two-way street.

Case study in dissemination for health policy

Case study: The NHS Next Stage Review: disseminating a vision for primary and community care in Britain

In July 2008 Britain's NHS published a report providing a new vision for how primary and community care services in that country could evolve over the next decade in ways characterized by continuous improvement, guaranteed essential standards, and reward for excellence. The vision was disseminated in a suite of related documents for different stakeholders. These extracted the key messages that the Department of Health and the NHS wanted stakeholders to know, including statements of what the vision means for the community, each tailor-made for particular stakeholders. Each of these tailor-made documents reiterated the key themes of the main report in relation to quality to help ensure shared understandings.[255] For example, the theme of integrated care was variously reiterated in statements and briefing papers for

- patients and the general public: how services will be connected in ways that save patients time and deliver them better care[270]
- the GP and practice staff: how better integrated care will work in practice for GPs and practice staff[271]
- nurses, midwives, and allied community health workers: how integrated clinical approaches and multi-professional engagement will give such community health workers a key role in influencing service transformation[272]
- local government staff: how councils as wider community agencies can work with health agencies to achieve integrated care in new settings.[273]

The NHS also used a wide range of formats designed to reach different audiences:

- a 'blog' site so that members of the community could ask questions directly to the review's leader Lord Darzi, the health minister
- a scholarly paper in *The Lancet* also by Lord Darzi[274]
- events in high profile locations where the report was launched
- a highly innovative 'virtual brochure' version of the Next Stage Review final report, available online, which included a video introduction from Lord Darzi, and facility for reader interaction (http://www.ournhs.nhs.uk)
- presentation of the review information in 'Second Life' interactive online formats (http://www.flickr.com) as well as streaming website videos of such events to provide video and audio formats for dissemination, including on YouTube (http://www.youtube.com)
- thumbnail web interfaces to disseminate more complex information such as interactive maps offering information on developments in local or regional visions for the new directions in healthcare delivery
- resources other agencies could use to disseminate the report such as downloadable videos, slides, logos and artwork, keys facts, and useful 'core scripts' for explaining the review.

Further, the NHS developed clusters of different kinds of documents (for informing, for implementing etc.). For example, a series of implementation strategy and guideline documents, such as workforce strategy documents (http://www.ournhs.nhs.uk), were developed and made widely available.

It is important to note that each form of information developed by the NHS and linked government agencies was carefully designed to meet the needs not simply of particular stakeholders, but of those specific stakeholders at particular points in time in the development, dissemination, and implementation of the review. This included showcasing information about the review on different kinds of government websites from the prime minister's website (http://www.number10.gov.uk) to the websites of local agencies, networks, and trusts linked to the NHS which also had a role in collecting information at the regional level (http://www.tin.nhs.uk). These agencies further translated the information about the review in, for example, summary reports for their board meetings and so on (http://www.stpct.nhs.uk).

At different stages of the consultations, after the review was completed, and sometimes as part of the process of implementation, many diverse agencies outside the NHS itself took a role in disseminating and translating the message of integration to the general public as well as specific stakeholder groups (professional, charitable, staff union, health industry, health and social services, voluntary community agencies, general and specialist library and online bookstores and public information agencies, universities and health research observatories, health journals, and non-university research and healthcare advocacy agencies). This took place, for example, for

- health agency leaders through information such as news bulletins on how integrated care will work at the broad system-wide level and why it is consistent with management needs[275] as well as specific health industry advocacy agencies (http://www.bivda.co.uk)

- specific groups of health professionals such as surgeons and physiotherapists through interpretation and debate including in journals[276](http://www.rcseng.ac.uk) (http://www.csp.org.uk)

- specific groups characterized by a particular condition such as arthritis through the advocacy work of specific groups (http://www.arthritiscare.org.uk), including groups defined by a particular geographic locale such as rural communities (http://www.ruralcommunities.gov.uk)

- the general public through charitable foundations organizing briefing papers and public debates (http://www.kingsfund.org.uk), including through a range of libraries and information centres (http://fadelibrary.wordpress.com)

Most of these disseminating organizations did not take a strong advocacy role that worked against the messages the NHS was trying to send about the review, including at the consultation stage. However, a series of carefully orchestrated media releases, including about the process of consultation at the local community or regional level, report launch events and media hotlines, were included in the media dissemination campaign (http://www.ournhs.nhs.uk). These did not prevent the review from receiving some strong criticism in, for example, the alternative press such as *Parliamentary Brief*, an independent commentary on British political affairs:

> The secretary of state is reported as saying at the launch of the Darzi NHS Next Stage review that it was based on 'evidence of good practice'. The political use of the word 'evidence' is increasingly a synonym for faith-based policy-making.
>
> Inevitably, one has sympathy for Darzi. General election fever led to the precipitate publication of half-baked proposals. (http://www.parliamentarybrief.com)

Generally speaking though, the media were favourable to the review, with limited discussion of opposing views of the review in newspapers such as the UK's influential Guardian.[277]

Appendix

CEO interview questions

1 Can you give some practical examples of how decisions are made about policy—what influences these decisions? What role does research have in policy-making?

2 Can you describe the features of a research report that really met the needs of health policy decision-making? What was it about that report that worked for health policy decision-making?

3 What's the best way for researchers to find out about the policy challenges they need to address in their research?

4 What do researchers need to cover when they do literature reviews for policy decision-makers?

5 What practical advice can you give to researchers about how to make their research methods more relevant to your needs? Are there any research techniques that you find especially persuasive and/or have currency in your policy-making circles?

6 How should researchers work with community stakeholders to make their research effective for policy-makers?

7 Can you describe the outputs of data analyses (graphs, tables, narrative analyses etc.) that have/haven't worked for the practical needs of policy decision-making? How should researchers create a policy story that weaves their data together to make a persuasive policy argument?

8 How should researchers write health policy options and recommendations that work for you?

9 What practical tips would you give researchers to help them make sure their research doesn't sit on a shelf gathering dust, but rather gets used by policy-makers and their communities?

References

1 Walker W, Harremoes P, Rotmans J et al. Defining uncertainty: a conceptual basis for uncertainty management in model-based decision support. *Integrated Assessment* 2003; 4(1): 5–17.

2 Lavis JN, Ross SE, Hurley JE. Examining the Role of Health Services Research in Public Policymaking doi:10.1111/1468-0009.00005. *The Milbank Quarterly* 2002; 80(1): 125–54.

3 Dubnick M, Bardes B. *Thinking about Public Policy: A Problem-Solving Approach*. New York, Wiley, 1983.

4 Hanney S, Gonzalez-Block M, Buxton M, Kogan M. The utilisation of health research in policy-making: concepts, examples and methods of assessment. *Health Research Policy and Systems* 2003; 1(2).

5 Duncan B. Health policy in the European Union: how it's made and how to influence it. *BMJ* 2002; 324(7344): 1027–30.

6 Elliott H, Popay J. How are policy makers using evidence? Models of research utilisation and local NHS policy making. *Journal of Epidemiology and Community Health* 2000; 54(6): 461–8.

7 Wildavsky A. *Speaking Truth to Power: the Art and Craft of Policy Analysis*. USA, Transaction Publishers, 1987.

8 Weiss C. The many meanings of research utilisation. *Public Administration Review* 1979; 39(5): 426–31.

9 Nutley S, Webb J. Evidence and the policy process. In: (eds). *What Works? Evidence Based Policy and Practice in Public Services*. Bristol: The Policy Press; 2000: pp. 13–41.

10 Willison DJ, MacLeod SM. The role of research evidence in pharmaceutical policy making: evidence when necessary but not necessarily evidence. *Journal of Evaluation in Clinical Practice* 1999; 5(2): 243–9.

11 Kay A. The abolition of the GP fundholding scheme: a lesson in evidence-based policy making. *British Journal of General Practice* 2002; (Feb): 141–4.

12 Hall P, Land H, Parker R, Webb A. *Change, Choice, and Conflict in Social Policy*. London, Heinemann, 1975.

13 Saltman R, Ferroussier-Davis O. The concept of stewardship in health policy. *Bulletin of the World Health Organisation* 2000; 78(6): 6–739.

14 Bullock H, Mountford J, Stanley R. *Better Policy-Making*. London, Centre for Management and Policy Studies, Cabinet Office, 2001.

15 Mechanic D. *The Truth about Health Care: Why Reform is not Working in America*. New Brunswick, Rutgers University Press, 2006.

16 Majone G. *Evidence, Argument & Persuasion in the Policy Process*. USA, Yale University Press, 1989.

17 Michaels S, Goucher NP, McCarthy D. Policy windows, policy change, and organizational learning: watersheds in the evolution of watershed management. *Environ Manage* 2006; 38(6): 983–92.

18 Mulgan G, Lee A. *Better Policy Delivery and Design: A Discussion Paper*. London, Cabinet Office, 2001.

19 Dobbins M, Jack S, Thomas H, Kothari A. Public health decision-makers' informational needs and preferences for receiving research evidence. *Worldviews on Evidence-Based Nursing* 2007; 4(3): 156–63.

20 Mays N, Pope C, Popay J. Systematically reviewing qualitative and quantitative evidence to inform management and policy-making in the health field. *Journal of Health Services Research & Policy* 2005; 10 (Suppl 1): 6–20.

21 Davies H, Nutley S, Smith P. Introducing evidence-based policy and practice in public services. In: (eds). *What Works? Evidence Based Policy and Practice in Public Services* Bristol: The Policy Press; 2000: pp. 1–11.

22 Palmer GR. Evidence-based health policy-making, hospital funding and health insurance. *Medical Journal of Australia* 2000; 172(3): 130–3.

23 Sorian R, Baugh T. The power of information: closing the gap between research and policy. *Health Affairs: The Policy Journal of the Health Sphere* 2002; 21(2): 264–73.

24 Dobbins M, Rosenbaum P, Plews N, et al. Information Transfer: What do decision-makers want and need from researchers?. *Implementation Science* 2007; 2(1): 20.

25 Weatherly H, Drummond M, Smith D. Using evidence in the development of local health policies. Some evidence from the United Kingdom. *International Journal of Technology Assessment in Health Care* 2002; 18(4): 771–81.

26 Oxman AD, Lavis JN, Fretheim A. Use of evidence in WHO recommendations. *Lancet* 2007; 369(9576): 1883–9.

27 Dobbins M, Cockerill R, Barnsley J. Factors affecting the utilization of systematic reviews: a study of public health decision makers. *International Journal of Technology Assessment in Health Care* 2001; 17(02): 203–14.

28 Dobbins M, Cockerill R, Barnsley J, Ciliska D. Factors of the innovation, organization, environment, and individual that predict the influence five systematic reviews had on public health decisions. *International Journal of Technology Assessment in Health Care* 2001; 17(4): 467–78.

29 Weissert C, Weissert W. *Governing Health: The Politics of Health Policy*. Baltimore, USA, The Johns Hopkins University Press, 2006.

30 Hoffmann C, Graf von der Schulenburg JM. The influence of economic evaluation studies on decision making. A European survey. The EUROMET group. *Health Policy* 2000; 52(3): 179–92.

31 Al MJ, Feenstra T, Brouwer WB. Decision makers' views on health care objectives and budget constraints: results from a pilot study. *Health Policy* 2004; 70(1): 33–48.

32 Kuruvilla S, Mays N, Walt G. Describing the impact of health services and policy research. *Journal of Health Services Research & Policy* 2007; 12 (Suppl 1): S1-23–31.

33 Bensing JM, Caris-Verhallen WM, Dekker J, Delnoij DM, et al. Doing the right thing and doing it right: toward a framework for assessing the policy relevance of health services research. *International Journal of Technology Assessment in Health Care* 2003; 19(4): 604–12.

34 Dobrow MJ, Goel V, Upshur REG. Evidence-based health policy: context and utilisation. *Social Science & Medicine* 2004; 58(1): 207–17.

35 Knott J, Wildavsky A. If dissemination is the solution, what is the problem?. *Knowledge: creation, diffusion, utilisation* 1980; 1: 537–78.

36 Nutley S, Walter I, Davies H. *Using Evidence: How Research can Inform Public Services*. Bristol, The Policy Press, 2007.

37 Smith KE. Health inequalities in Scotland and England: the contrasting journeys of ideas from research into policy. *Social Science & Medicine* 2007; 64(7): 1438–49.

38 Kindig D, Day P, Fox DM, et al. What new knowledge would help policymakers better balance investments for optimal health outcomes? *Health Services Research* 2003; 38(6 Pt 2): 1923–38.

39 Davey Smith G, Ebrahim S, Frankel S. How policy informs the evidence: "evidence based" thinking can lead to debased policy making. *British Medical Journal* 2001; 322(7280): 184–5.

40 Kemm J. The limitations of 'evidence-based' public health. *Journal of Evaluation in Clinical Practice* 2006; 12(3): 319–24.

41 Smith-Merry J, Gillespie J, Leeder SR. A pathway to a stronger research culture in health policy. *Australia and New Zealand Health Policy* 2007; 4: 19.

42 Ball A. *Education reform: a critical and post-structural approach*. Buckingham, UK, Open University Press, 1994.

43 Gale T. Policy trajectories: treading the discursive path of policy analysis. *Discourse: Studies in the Cultural Politics of Education* 1999; 20(3): 393–407.

44 Strategic Policy Making Team. *Professional Policy Making for the 21st Century: version 2*. Cabinet Office, 1999.

45 Black N. Evidence-based policy: proceed with care. *British Medical Journal* 2001; 323(7307): 275–9.

46 Corrigan P, Watson A. Factors that explain how policy makers distribute resources to mental health services. *Psychiatric Services* 2003; 54: 501–7.

47 Lavis J, Farrant M, Stoddart G. Barriers to employment-related healthy public policy in Canada. *Health Promotion International* 2001; 16(1): 9–20.

48 Lin V. From public health research to health promotion policy: On the 10 major contradictions. *Sozial- und Praventivmedizin* 2004; 49(3): 179–84.

49 Innvaer S, Vist G, Trommald M, Oxman A. Health policy-makers' perceptions of their use of evidence: a systematic review. *Journal of Health Services Research & Policy* 2002; 7(4): 239–44.

50 Nutley S, Walter I, Davies H. *Using Evidence: How Research Can Inform Public Services*. Bristol, The Policy Press, 2007.

51 Davenport C, Mathers J, Parry J. Use of health impact assessment in incorporating health considerations in decision making. *Journal of Epidemiology and Community Health* 2006; 60(3): 196–201.

52 Petticrew M, Whitehead M, Macintyre S, et al. Evidence for public health policy on inequalities: 1: the reality according to policy-makers. *Journal of Epidemiology and Community Health* 2004; 58: 811–6.

53 Ross S, Lavis J, Rodriguez C, et al. Partnership experiences: involving decision-makers in the research process. *Journal of Health Services Research & Policy* 2003; 8 (Suppl 2): 26–34.

54 Rosenstock L, Jackson Lee L. Attacks on science: the risks to evidence-based policy. *American Journal of Public Health* 2002; 92(1): 14–8.

55 King G, Gakidou E, Ravishankar N, et al. A "politically robust" experimental design for public policy evaluation, with application to the Mexican universal health insurance program. *Journal of Policy Analysis and Management* 2007; 26(3): 479–506.

56 Birnbaum R. Policy Scholars Are from Venus; Policy Makers Are from Mars. *The Review of Higher Education* 2000; 23(2): 119–32.

57 Mitton C, Patten S. Evidence-based priority-setting: what do the decision-makers think?. *Journal of Health Services Research & Policy* 2004; 9(3): 146–52.

58 Ham C. Values and Health Policy: The Case of Singapore. *Journal of Health Politics Policy and Law* 2001; 26(4): 739–46.

59 Acheson D. *Independent Inquiry into Inequalities in Health*. London, Stationery Office, 1998.

60 Martin Laffin AT. New Labour and Government in Britain: Change or Continuity?. *Australian Journal of Public Administration* 1997; 56(4): 117–27.

61 Black D, Morris J, Smith C, et al. *Inequalities in health: report of a research working group (Black report)*. London, Department of Health and Social Security, 1980.

62 Macintyre S, Chalmers I, Horton R, Smith R. Using evidence to inform health policy: case study. *British Medical Journal* 2001; 322(7280): 222–5.

63 Blane D. Health inequality and public policy: one year on from the Acheson report. *Journal of Epidemiology and Community Health* 1999; 53(12): 748.

64 Stiefel M, Rothert K, Crane R, et al. Kaiser Permanente's National Integrated Diabetes Care Management Program Informing Judgment: Case Studies of Health Policy and Research in Six Countries 2001 [online]. Milbank Memorial Fund. Available at: http://www.milbank.org/reports/2001cochrane/010903cochrane.html#foreword. Accessed 10 November, 2008

65 Dobrow MJ, Goel V, Lemieux-Charles L, Black NA. The impact of context on evidence utilization: a framework for expert groups developing health policy recommendations. *Social Science & Medicine* 2006; 63(7): 1811–24.

66 Waddell C. So much research evidence, so little dissemination and uptake: mixing the useful with the pleasing. *Evidence Based Mental Health* 2001; 4: 3–5.

67 Bowen S, Zwi A. Pathways to "Evidence-Informed" Policy and Practice: A Framework for Action. *PLoS Medicine* 2005; 2(7): 0600–5.

68 Bensing J, Caris-Verhallen W, Dekker J, et al. Doing the right thing and doing it right: toward a framework for assessing the policy relevance of health services research. *International Journal of Technology Assessment in Health Care* 2003; 19(4): 604–12.

69 Landry R, Lamari M, Amara N. The extent and determinants of the utilization of university research in government agencies. *Public Administration Review* 2003; 63(2): 192–205.

70 Smith C. *Writing Public Policy: A Practical Guide to Communicating in the Policy-Making Process*. Oxford, Oxford University Press, 2005.

71 Majone G. *Evidence, Argument & Persuasion in the Policy Process*. USA, Yale University Press, 1992.

72 HM Treasury. The Green Book: Appraisal and Evaluation in Central Government. u.d [online]. HM Treasury. Available at: http://www.hm-treasury.gov.uk/media/9/C/Green_Book_03.pdf. Accessed 21 May, 2008

73 Nelson D, Hess B, Croyle R. *Making Data Talk: The Science and Practice of Translating Public Health Research and Surveillance Findings to Policy Makers, the Public, and the Press*. USA, Oxford University Press, 2009.

74 Knoepfel P, Larrue C, Varone F, Hill M. *Public Policy Analysis*. Bristol, The Policy Press, 2007.

75 Department of Health. *Choosing Health: Making Healthy Choices Easier.* London, National Health Service, 2004.

76 Australian Department of Health and Ageing. *Report on the Audit of Health Workforce in Rural and Regional Australia.* Canberra, Commonwealth of Australia, 2008.

77 Australian Government Department of Health and Ageing. *Report on the Audit of Health Workforce in Rural and Regional Australia.* Canberra, Commonwealth of Australia, 2008.

78 Freeman R. Health policy and the problem of learning. 2000 [online]. School of Social and Political Studies, University of Edinburgh). Available at: http://64.233.179.104/scholar?hl=en&lr=&q=cache:qbxqvZARItQJ:www.pol.ed.ac.uk/freeman/workingpapers/healthpolicy_learning.pdf+how±to±write±for±±%22health±policy±makers%22. Accessed 13 September, 2007

79 Sheldon T. Learning from abroad or policy tourism?. *British Journal of General Practice* 2004; 54(503): 410–1.

80 Waters E, Doyle J, Jackson N, et al. Evaluating the effectiveness of public health interventions: the role and activities of the Cochrane Collaboration. *Journal of Epidemiology and Community Health* 2006; 60(4): 285–9.

81 Lavis J, Davies H, Oxman A, et al. Towards systematic reviews that inform health care management and policy-making. *Journal of Health Services Research & Policy* 2005; 10 (Suppl 1): 35–48.

82 Government Chief Social Researcher's Office. Magenta Book: Guidance Notes on Policy Evaluation. 1997 [online]. Cabinet Office. Available at: http://www.nationalschool.gov.uk/policyhub/magenta_book/index.asp. Accessed 21 May, 2008

83 Hall JG, Bainbridge L, Buchan A, et al. A meeting of minds: Interdisciplinary research in the health sciences in Canada. *Canadian Medical Association Journal* 2006; 175(7): 763–71.

84 Pawson R, Greenhalgh T, Harvey G, Walshe K. Realist review: a new method of systematic review designed for complex policy interventions. *Journal of Health Services Research & Policy* 2005; 10 (Suppl 1): 21–34.

85 McKinlay JB, Marceau LD. To boldly go. *American Journal of Public Health* 2000; 90(1): 25–33.

86 Mannion R, Goddard M. Performance measurement and improvement in health care. *Applied Health Economics and Health Policy* 2002; 1(1): 13–23.

87 Moynihan R. *Evaluating health services: a reporter covers the science of research synthesis.* New York, Milbank Memorial Fund, 2004.

88 Benzies KM, Premji S, Hayden KA, Serrett K. State-of-the-evidence reviews: Advantages and challenges of including grey literature. *Worldviews on Evidence-Based Nursing* 2006; 3(2): 55–61.

89 Mitchell J. Case and Situational Analysis. *Sociology Review* 1983; 31: 187–211.

90 Peck J. Fuzzy old world: A reponse to Markusen. *Regional Studies* 2003; 37(6–7): 729–40.

91 Gibbs GR, Hall C. The research potential of testimony from public inquiry websites. *Children and Society* 2007; 21(1): 69–79.

92 Popay J, Rogers A, Williams G. Rationale and Standards for the Systematic Review of Qualitative Literature in Health Services Research. *Qualitative Health Research* 1998; 8(3): 341–51.

93 Office of Management and Budget. What Constitutes Strong Evidence of a Program's Effectiveness? 2007? [online]. The Council for Excellence in Government. Available at: http://www.excelgov.org/index.php?keyword=a432fbc34d71c7. Accessed 19 May, 2008

94 Spencer L, Ritchie J, Lewis J, Dillon L. *Quality in Qualitative Evaluation: A Framework for Assessing Research Evidence*. London, Government Chief Social Researcher's Office, Cabinet Office, 2003.

95 Arksey H, O'Malley L. Scoping studies: Towards a methodological framework. *International Journal of Social Research Methodology: Theory and Practice* 2005; 8(1): 19–32.

96 Pawson R. *Evidence-Based Policy: A Realist Perspective*. Los Angeles, Sage Publications, 2006.

97 Noblit G, Hare R. *Meta-Ethnography: Synthesising Qualitative Studies*. Newbury Park, California, Sage Publications, Inc, 1988.

98 Egger M, Davey Smith G, Altman D, (Eds). *Systematic Reviews in Health Care: Meta-Analysis in Context*. London, BMJ Publishing Group, 2001.

99 Petrosino A, Boruch RF, Soydan H, et al. Meeting the Challenges of Evidence-Based Policy: The Campbell Collaboration. *The ANNALS of the American Academy of Political and Social Science* 2001; 578(1): 14–34.

100 Pawson R. Evidence-based Policy: In Search of a Method. *Evaluation* 2002; 8(2): 157–81.

101 Ministry of Health. *Communicable Disease Surveillance in Singapore 2007*. Singapore, Singapore Government, 2007.

102 National Preventative Health Taskforce. *Australia: The Healthiest Country by 2020 A Discussion Paper*. Canberra, Commonwealth of Australia, 2008.

103 Obesity Working Group for the National Preventative Taskforce. *Technical Report No 1 Obesity in Australia: A Need for Urgent Action*. Canberra, Commonwealth of Australia, 2008.

104 Tobacco Working Group for the National Preventative Health Taskforce. *Technical Report No 2 Tobacco Control in Australia: Making Smoking History*. Canberra, Commonwealth of Australia, 2008.

105 Alcohol Working Group for the National Preventative Health Taskforce. *Technical Report No 3 Preventing Alcohol-related Harm in Australia: A Window of Opportunity*. Canberra, Commonwealth of Australia, 2008.

106 Mercer SL, DeVinney BJ, Fine LJ, et al. Study Designs for Effectiveness and Translation Research. Identifying Trade-offs. *American Journal of Preventive Medicine* 2007; 33(2): 139–54.e2.

107 Fox NJ. Practice-based evidence: Towards collaborative and transgressive research. *Sociology* 2003; 37(1): 81–102.

108 Glasgow R, Magid D, Beck A, et al. Practical clinical trials for translating research to practice: design and measurement recommendations. *Medical Care* 2005; 43(6): 551–7.

109 Green LW, Glasgow RE. Evaluating the relevance, generalization, and applicability of research: Issues in external validation and translation methodology. *Evaluation and the Health Professions* 2006; 29(1): 126–53.

110   Lewis S. Toward a general theory of indifference to research-based evidence. *Journal of Health Services Research & Policy* 2007; 12(3): 166–72.

111   Davies H, Nutley S. Healthcare: evidence to the fore. In: (eds). *What Works? Evidence Based Policy and Practice in Public Services.* Bristol: The Policy Press; 2000: pp. 43–67.

112   Macintyre S, Petticrew M. Good intentions and received wisdom are not enough. *Journal of Epidemiology and Community Health* 2000; 54(11): 802–3.

113   Goodacre S. Research methods: Beyond the clinical trial. *Annals of Emergency Medicine* 2003; 42(1): 56–65.

114   Tunis SR, Stryer DB, Clancy CM. Practical clinical trials: increasing the value of clinical research for decision making in clinical and health policy. *Jama* 2003; 290(12): 1624–32.

115   Jack SM. Utility of qualitative research findings in evidence-based public health practice. *Public Health Nursing* 2006; 23(3): 277–83.

116   Rothstein H, Tonges MC. Beyond the significance test in administrative research and policy decisions. *Journal of Nursing Scholarship* 2000; 32(1): 65–70.

117   Gilbert N. Simulation: A new way of doing social science. *American Behavioral Scientist* 1999; 42(10): 1485–7.

118   Weinstein MC, Toy EL, Sandberg EA, et al. Modeling for health care and other policy decisions: Uses, roles, and validity. *Value in Health* 2001; 4(5): 348–61.

119   Nuijten M, Starzewski J. Applications of modelling studies. *Pharmacoeconomics* 1998; 13(3): 289–91.

120   Brandt PT, Freeman JR. Advances in Bayesian time series modeling and the study of politics: Theory testing, forecasting, and policy analysis. *Political Analysis* 2006; 14(1): 1–36.

121   Weinstein MC, O'Brien B, Hornberger J, et al. Principles of good practice for decision analytic modeling in health-care evaluation: Report of the ISPOR task force on good research practices - Modeling studies. *Value in Health* 2003; 6(1): 9–17.

122   Kaplan EH. Adventures in policy modeling! Operations research in the community and beyond. *Omega* 2008; 36(1): 1–9.

123   Royston G, Halsall J, Halsall D, Braithwaite C. Operational research for informed innovation: NHS Direct as a case study in the design, implementation and evaluation of a new public service. *Journal of the Operational Research Society* 2003; 54(10): 1022–8.

124   Gallivan S. Mathematical methods to assist with hospital operation and planning. *Clinical and Investigative Medicine* 2005; 28(6): 326–30.

125   Codrington-Virtue A, Chaussalet T, Whittlestone P, Kelly J. Developing an application of and accident and emergency patient simulation In: Brialsford S, Harper P, (eds). *Operational Research for Health Policy: Making Better Decisions; 31st Annual Conference of the European Working Group on Operational Research Applied to Health Services, Southampton, UK, 2007.* Peter Lang.

126   White L. The Role of Systems Research and Operational Research in Community Involvement: A Case Study of a Health Action Zone. *Systems Research and Behavioral Science* 2003; 20(2): 133–45.

127   Brandeau M, Sainfort F, Pierskalla W. *Operations Research and Health Care: A Handbook of Methods and Applications.* Boston, Kluwer Academic Publishers, 2004.

128 Hillier F, Lieberman G. *Introduction to Operations Research.* Boston, McGrawHill Higher Education, 2005.

129 Provan K, Milward H. A preliminary theory of interorganisational network effectiveness: a comparative study of four community mental health systems. *Administrative Science Quarterly* 1995; 40: 1–33.

130 Berry FS, Brower RS, Choi SO, et al. Three traditions of network research: What the public management research agenda can learn from other research communities. *Public Administration Review* 2004; 64(5): 539–52.

131 Huang CY, Sun CT, Hsieh JL, Lin H. Simulating SARS: Small-World Epidemiological Modeling and Public Health Policy Assessments. *Journal of Artificial Societies and Social Simulation* 2004; 7(4): http://jasss.soc.surrey.ac.uk/7/4/2.html.

132 Morrato EH, Elias M, Gericke CA. Using population-based routine data for evidence-based health policy decisions: lessons from three examples of setting and evaluating national health policy in Australia, the UK and the USA. *Journal of Public Health (Oxf)* 2007; 29(4): 463–71.

133 Gerrish K. Researching ethnic diversity in the British NHS: Methodological and practical concerns. *Journal of Advanced Nursing* 2000; 31(4): 918–25.

134 Attia J, Page J, Heller RF, Dobson AJ. Impact numbers in health policy decisions. *Journal of Epidemiology and Community Health* 2002; 56(8): 600–5.

135 Hoffman C, Stoykova B, Nixon J, et al. Do health-care decision makers find economic evaluations useful? The findings of focus group research in UK health authorities. *Value Health* 2002; 5(2): 71–8.

136 Noyes K, Holloway RG. Evidence from Cost-Effectiveness Research. *NeuroRx* 2004; 1(3): 348–55.

137 Jack W. Public spending on health care: how are different criteria related? A second opinion. *Health Policy* 2000; 53(1): 61–7.

138 Cooper NJ, Sutton AJ, Abrams KR, et al. Comprehensive decision analytical modelling in economic evaluation: A Bayesian approach. *Health Economics* 2004; 13(3): 203–6.

139 Fenwick E, Claxton K, Sculpher M. Representing uncertainty: The role of cost-effectiveness acceptability curves. *Health Economics* 2001; 10(8): 779–87.

140 Mauskopf J, Paul J, Grant D, Stergachis A. The role of cost-consequence analysis in healthcare decision-making. *Pharmacoeconomics* 1998; 13(3): 277–88.

141 Ubel PA, Hirth RA, Chernew ME, Fendrick AM. What is the price of life and why doesn't it increase at the rate of inflation?. *Archives of Internal Medicine* 2003; 163(14): 1637–41.

142 Neumann PJ, Goldie SJ, Weinstein MC. Preference-based measures in economic evaluation in health care. *Annual Review of Public Health* 2000; 21: 587–611.

143 Ramsey SD, McIntosh M, Sullivan SD. Design issues for conducting cost-effectiveness analyses alongside clinical trials. *Annual Review of Public Health* 2001; 22: 129–41.

144 The Comptroller and Auditor General. *Modern Policy-Making: Ensuring Policies Deliver Value for Money.* London, Stationery Office, 2001.

145 Kane NM, Magnus SA. The Medicare Cost Report and the limits of hospital accountability: improving financial accounting data. *Journal of Health Politics, Policy and Law* 2001; 26(1): 81–105.

146 Wells R, Banaszak-Holl J. A critical review of recent US market level health care strategy literature. *Social Science & Medicine* 2000; 51(5): 639–56.

147 Meltzer D, Chung J. Effects of competition under prospective payment on hospital costs. In: Garber A, (ed.), *Frontiers in Health Policy Research*, Bethesda, Maryland, 2001. MIT Press.

148 Sloan F. Frontiers in Health Policy Research. In: Garber A, (ed.), Bethesda, Maryland, 2001. MIT Press.

149 Marmor T. *Fads, Fallacies and Foolishness in Medical Care Management and Policy*. Hackensack, New Jersey, World Scientific, 2007.

150 Beynon M, Kitchener M. Ranking the 'balance' of state long-term care systems: a comparative exposition of the SMARTER and CaRBS techniques. *Health Care Management Science* 2005; 8: 157–66.

151 Murphy E, Dingwell R. *Qualitative Methods and Health Policy Research*. New York, Walter de Gruyter, Inc, 2003.

152 Davies P. Contributions from qualitative research. In: Davies H, Nutley S, Smith P (eds). *What Works? Evidence Based Policy and Practice in Public Services*. Bristol: The Policy Press; 2000: pp. 291–396.

153 Sofaer S. Qualitative methods: what are they and why use them?. *Health Services Research* 1999; 34(5 Pt 2): 1101–18.

154 Ryan P. The policy sciences and the unmasking turn of mind. *Review of Policy Research* 2004; 21(5): 715–28.

155 Stone D. *Policy Paradox: The Art of Political Decision-Making*. New York, W.W. Norton, 2002.

156 Foucault M. *Discipline and Punish: The Birth of the Prison*. Harmondsworth, Penguin, 1977.

157 Martin D, Singer P. A strategy to improve priority setting in health care institutions. *Health Care Anal* 2003; 11(1): 59–68.

158 Daniels N, Sabin J. *Setting Limits Fairly: Can we Learn to Share Medical Resources?*. Oxford, Oxford University Press, 2002.

159 Fairclough N. *Discourse and social change*. Cambridge, Polity Press, 1992.

160 Fairclough N. *Critical discourse analysis*. London, Longman, 1995.

161 Ragin C. *Fuzzy-Set Social Science*. Chicago, The University of Chicago Press, 2000.

162 Grosskurth J, Rotmans J. The SCENE model: getting a grip on sustainable development in policy making. *Environment, Development and Sustainability* 2005; 7: 135–51.

163 Busse R, Schlette S, Weinbrenner S, (Eds). *Health Policy Developments: Issue 4; Focus on Access, Primary Care, Health Care Organisation*. Gutersloh, Germany, Verlag Bertelsmann Stiftung, 2005.

164 Fontela E. The future societal bill: Methodological alternatives. *Futures* 2003; 35(1): 25–36.

165 Séguin J, (Ed.). *Human Health in a Changing Climate: A Canadian Assessment of Vulnerabilities and Adaptive Capacity*. Ottawa, Canada, Health Canada, 2008.

166 Department of Health and Ageing. *The State of our Public Hospitals: June 2008 Report*. Canberra, Commonwealth of Australia, 2008.

167 Rosenbach M, Irvin C, Merrill A, et al. *National Evaluation of the State Children's Health Insurance Program: A Decade of Expanding Coverage and Improving Access: Final Report*. Cambridge, MA, Mathematica Policy Research, Inc., 2007.

168 Department of Health Statistics and Informatics. *The Global Burden of Disease 2004 Update*. Geneva, Information, Evidence and Research Cluster, World Health Organisation, 2008.

169 Jobes PC, Barclay E, Donnermeyer JF. Preaching to the choir: A comparison of the use of integrated data sets in criminology journals in Australia, England and the United States. *Australian and New Zealand Journal of Criminology* 2002; 35(1): 79–98.

170 McCann M. Causal versus constitutive explanations (or, on the difficulty of being so positive . . .). *Law and Social Inquiry* 1996; 21(2): 457–81.

171 Goldstone JA, Useem B. Prison riots as microrevolutions: An extension of state-centered theories of revolution. *American Journal of Sociology* 1999; 10(4): 985–1029.

172 Mahoney J. Nominal, ordinal, and narrative appraisal in macrocausal analysis. *American Journal of Sociology* 1999; 10(4): 1154–96.

173 Yamaguchi K. Mathematical sociology and empirical research. *Sociological Theory and Methods* 2005; 20(2): 137–56.

174 George A, Bennett A. *Case Studies and Theory Development in the Social Sciences*. Cambridge, MA, MIT Press, 2005.

175 Pawson R, Tilley N. *Realistic Evaluation*. London, Sage Publications, 2000.

176 Ragin CC. Using qualitative comparative analysis to study causal complexity. *Health Services Research* 1999; 34(5 Part II): 1225–39.

177 Ragin CC. The distinctiveness of case-oriented research. *Health Services Research* 1999; 34(5 Part II): 1137–51.

178 Bell E. Quali-Quantitative Analysis: Why it could open new frontiers for holistic health practice [paper presented at the 3rd International Conference on Holistic Health in Copenhagen, Denmark, 17–18 November 2006]. *The Scientific World: Holistic Health & Medicine* 2006; 1: 321–31.

179 Bell E. Time, space, and body in adolescent residential services: re-imagining service design research. *Addiction Theory and Research* 2007; 15(11): 85–9.

180 Bell E. Quali-Quantitative Analysis: A new model for evaluation of unusual cases in hospital performance?. *Australian Health Review* 2006; 31 (Suppl.1): S86–S97.

181 Ragin C. *The Comparative Method*. Los Angeles, University of California Press, 1987.

182 Ragin C. Using qualitative comparative analysis to study configurations. In: Kelle U (eds). *Computer-Aided Qualitative Data Analysis: Theory, Methods and Practice*. London: SAGE Publications; 1995: pp.

183 Ragin C. Turning the tables: How case-oriented research challenges variable-oriented research. *Comparative Social Research* 1997; 16: 27–42.

184 Ragin CC. Fuzzy-Set Analysis of Necessary Conditions. In: Goertz G, Starr H (eds). *Necessary Conditions: Theory, Methodology and Applications*. Lanham, Maryland: Rowman and Littleford; 2002: pp. 179–196.

185 Ragin C, Drass K, Davey S. *Fuzzy-Set/Qualitative Comparative Analysis 2.0*. Tucson, Arizona, Department of Sociology, University of Arizona, 2006.

186 Rihoux B, Ragin C (Eds). *Configurational Comparative Methods: Qualitative Comparative Analysis (QCA) and Related Techniques*. Los Angeles, Sage, 2009.

187 Bell E, Hall R. 'Dead in the water': Is rural violent crime prevention floating face-down because criminology can't handle context?. *Crime Prevention & Community Safety* 2007; 9 (4): doi:10.1057/palgrave.cpcs.8150051.

188 De Meur G, Rihoux B. *L'Analyse Quali-Quantitative Comparee (AQQC-QCA): Approche, Techniques et applications en sciences humanines:*. Louvain-La-Neuve, Belgium, Academia Bruylant, 2002.

189 Derrida J. *Speech and Phenomena and Other Essays on Husserl's Theory of Signs.* Evanston, Northwestern University Press, 1973.

190 Derrida J. *Of Grammatology.* Baltimore, Johns Hopkins University Press, 1976.

191 Derrida J. *Writing and Difference.* Chicago, University of Chicago Press, 1978.

192 Ragin C. Set relations in social research: evaluating their consistency and coverage. *Political Analysis* 2006; 14(3): 291–310.

193 Ragin C. The limitations of net effects in thinking. In: Grimm H, Rihoux B (eds). *Innovative Comparative Methods for Policy Analysis.* New York: Springer; 2006: pp. 13–41.

194 Gillespie L, Gillespie W, Robertson M, Lamb S, et al. Interventions for preventing falls in elderly people. *The Cochrane Database of Systematic Reviews* 2003; (4): Art. No.: CD000340. DOI: 10.1002/14651858.CD000340.

195 Li F, Fisher K, Harmer P, et al. Fear of falling in elderly persons: association with falls, functional ability, and quality of life. *The Journals of Gerontology Series B: Psychological Sciences and Social Sciences* 2003; 58: 283–90.

196 Alpini D, Cesarani A, Pugnetti L, et al. Project to prevent mobility-related accidents in elderly and disables. *The 3rd European Conference on Disability, Virtual Reality and Associated Technologies*, Italy, 2000. University of Reading.

197 Swift C. Care of older people: falls in late life and their consequences-implementing effective services. *British Medical Journal* 2001; 322: 855–7.

198 Khan K, Liu-Ambrose T, Donaldson M, McKay H. Physical activity to prevent falls in older people: time to intervene in high risk groups using falls as an outcome. *British Journal of Sports Medicine* 2001; 35: 144–5.

199 Hill H, Schwarz J. Assessment and management of falls in older people. *Internal Medicine Journal* 2004; 34: 557–64.

200 Theodos P. Fall prevention in frail elderly nursing home residents: a challenge to case management: part 1. *Lippincott's Case Management* 2003; 8(6): 246–51.

201 Menz H, Lord S. Foot problems, functional impairment, and falls in older people. *Journal of the American Podiatric Medical Association* 1999; 89(9): 458–67.

202 Li F, Harmer P, Fisher K, McAuley E. Tai chi: improving functional balance and predicting subsequent falls in older persons. *Medicine & Science in Sports & Exercise* 2004; 36(12): 2046–52.

203 Steadman J, Donaldson N, Kalra L. A randomized controlled trial of an enhanced balance training program to improve mobility and reduce falls in elderly patients. *Journal of the American Geriatrics Society* 2003; 51(6): 847–52.

204 Capezuti E. Building the science of falls-prevention research. *Journal of the American Geriatrics Society* 2004; 52(3): 461–2.

205 Weiss C, Holland E, Cable G, Ellison C, et al. An intervention to prevent falls in the elderly: a time series quasiexperiment. *Clinical Excellence for Nurse Practitioners* 2002; 6(3): 55–60.

206 Steinberg PF. Causal assessment in small-N policy studies. *Policy Studies Journal* 2007; 35(2): 181–204.

207 Young AF, Chesson RA. Obtaining views on health care from people with learning disabilities and severe mental health problems. *British Journal of Learning Disabilities* 2006; 34(1): 11–9.

208 Cabinet Office. *Modernising Government.* London, Stationery Office, 1999.

209 Barber R, Boote JD, Cooper CL. Involving consumers successfully in NHS research: a national survey. *Health Expect* 2007; 10(4): 380–91.

210 Wagle U. The policy science of democracy: The issues of methodology and citizen participation. *Policy Sciences* 2000; 33(2): 207–23.

211 Smith J, Prideaux D, Wolfe C, et al. Developing the accredited postgraduate assessment program for Fellowship of the Australian College of Rural and Remote medicine. *Rural and Remote Health* 2007; 7(805): online http://www.rrh.org.au.

212 Levitt M. Public consultation in bioethics. What's the point of asking the public when they have neither scientific nor ethical expertise? *Health Care Analysis* 2003; 11(1): 15–25.

213 Burgess J. Follow the argument where it leads: some personal reflections on 'policy-relevant' research. *Transactions of the Institute of British Geographers* 2005; 30(3): 273–81.

214 de Leeuw E. Investigating policy networks for health: theory and method in a larger organisational perspective. *World Health Organisational Regional Publications: European Series* 2001; 92: 185–206.

215 White L, Taket A. Beyond appraisal: participatory appraisal of needs and the development of action (PANDA). *Omega: International Journal of Management Science* 1997; 25(5): 523–35.

216 Cabinet Office. *Viewfinder: A Policy Maker's Guide to Public Involvement.* London, UK Government.

217 Arnstein S. A ladder of citizen participation in the USA. *Journal of American Institute of Planners* 1969; 35(4): 214–24.

218 Ellis G, Barry J, Robinson C. Many ways to say 'no', different ways to say 'yes': Applying Q-Methodology to understand public acceptance of wind farm proposals. *Journal of Environmental Planning and Management* 2007; 50(4): 517–51.

219 Gusfield J. *The culture of public problems: drinking-driving and the symbolic order.* Chicago, University of Chicago Press, 1981.

220 Kenny N, Giacomini M. Wanted: A new ethics field for health policy analysis. *Health Care Analysis* 2005; 13(4): 247–60.

221 Salmon A. Walking the talk: How participatory interview methods can democratize research. *Qualitative Health Research* 2007; 17(7): 982–93.

222 National Health and Medical Research Council. *Values and Ethics: Guidelines for Ethiccal Conduct in Aboriginal and Torres Strait Islander Research.* Canberra, National Health and Medical Research Council, 2003.

223 Minkler M, wallerstein N, (Eds). *Community Based Participatory Research for Health.* San Francisco, Jossey-Bass, 2003.

224 Gramberger M. *Citizens as Partners: OECD Handbook on Information, Consultation and Public Participation in Policy-Making.* Paris, Organisation for Economic Co-operation and Development, 2001.

225 Farrell C. *Patient and Public Involvement in Health: The Evidence for Policy Implementation: A Summary of the Results of the Health in Partnership Research Programme.* London, Department of Health, 2004.

226 Health Canada. *Health Canada Policy Toolkit for Public Involvement in Decision Making*. Ottawa, Ontario, Health Canada, 2000.

227 Ross F, Donovan S, Brearley S, et al. Involving older people in research: methodological issues. *Health & Social Care in the Community* 2005; 13(3): 268–75.

228 Minkler M, Vasquez VB, Warner JR, et al. Sowing the seeds for sustainable change: a community-based participatory research partnership for health promotion in Indiana, USA and its aftermath. *Health Promotion International* 2006; 21(4): 293–300.

229 Taket A, White L. Experience in the practice of one tradition of multimethodology. *Systems Practice and Action Research* 1998; 11(2): 153–68.

230 White L, Taket A, Gibbons M. *Working with Groups: Field Work Manual, Version 1.0.* London, South Bank University, 1996.

231 VanGeest JB, Johnson TP, Welch VL. Methodologies for improving response rates in surveys of physicians: A systematic review. *Evaluation and the Health Professions* 2007; 30(4): 303–21.

232 O'Fallon LR, Wolfle GM, Brown D, et al. Strategies for setting a national research agenda that is responsive to community needs. *Environmental Health Perspectives* 2003; 111(16): 1855–60.

233 Franklin KK, Hart JK. Idea generation and exploration: Benefits and limitations of the policy delphi research method. *Innovative Higher Education* 2007; 31(4): 237–46.

234 Nakash RA, Hutton JL, Jorstad-Stein EC, ct al. Maximising response to postal questionnaires–a systematic review of randomised trials in health research. *BMC Medical Research Methodology* 2006; 6: 5.

235 Nilsen ES, Myrhaug HT, Johansen M, et al. Methods of consumer involvement in developing healthcare policy and research, clinical practice guidelines and patient information material. *Cochrane Database Syst Rev* 2006; 3: CD004563.

236 Abelson J, Forest PG, Eyles J, et al. Will it make a difference if I show up and share? A citizens' perspective on improving public involvement processes for health system decision-making. *Journal of Health Services Research and Policy* 2004; 9(4): 205–12.

237 National Health Services. *Our Health, Our Care, Our Say*. London, National Health Services, 2006.

238 Department of Health. *Independence, Well-being and Choice: Our Vision for the Future of Social Care for Adults in England*. London, The Stationery Office, 2005.

239 Department of Health. *Responses to the Consultation on Adult Social Care in England: Analysis of Feedback from the Green Paper Independence, Well-being and Choice*. London, Department of Health, 2005.

240 Hastings A. Connecting Linguistic Structures and Social Practices: a Discursive Approach to Social Policy Analysis. *Journal of Social Policy* 1998; 27: 191–211.

241 Stone D. Causal stories and the formation of policy agendas. *Political Science Quarterly* 1989; 104: 281–300.

242 Porter T. *Trust in Numbers: The Pursuit of Objectivity in Science and Public Life*. Princeton, Princeton University Press, 1995.

243 McDonough J. Using and misusing anecdote in policy making. *Health Affairs: The Policy Journal of the Health Sphere* 2001; 20(1): 207–12.

244 Enkin M, Jadad A. Using anecdotal information in evidence-based health care: heresy or necessity?. *Annals of Oncology* 1998; 9: 963–6.

245 Veugelers PJ, Hornibrook S. Small area comparisons of health: applications for policy makers and challenges for researchers. *Chronic Dis Can* 2002; 23(3): 100–10.

246 Iser W. *The Implied Reader: Patterns of Communication in Prose Fiction from Bunyan to Beckett*. Baltimore, USA, The Johns Hopkins University Press, 1974.

247 Strunk W, White E. *The Elements of Style*. Massachusetts, Pearson Education Company, 2000.

248 Evans RG, Stoddart GL. Consuming Research, Producing Policy?. *American Journal of Public Health* 2003; 93(3): 371–9.

249 Smith G, Norris J, Shaw M. The independent inquiry into inequalities in health is welcome, but its recommendations are too cautious and vague. *British Medical Journal* 1998; 317(7171): 1465–6.

250 Acheson D, Baker D, Illsley R. Inequalities in health. *British Medical Journal* 1998; 317(7173): 1659–.

251 Poynor R. *No More Rules: Graphic Design and Postmodernism*. New Haven, Yale University Press, 2003.

252 Ministry of Health Welfare and Sport. *Policy for Older Persons in the Perspective of an Ageing Population*. The Hague, Ministry of Health, Welfare and Sport, 2006.

253 Department of Health & Children. *Building a Culture of Patient Safety and Quality Assurance*. Dublin, The Stationery Office, 2008.

254 Dr Foster Intelligence. *Hospital Guide 2008: The Health of our Hospitals Revealed*. London, Dr Foster Intelligence, 2008.

255 Lord Darzi. *High Quality Care for All: NHS Next Stage Review Final Report*. London, Department of Health, National Health Service 2008.

256 Mindell J, McKee M. Hospital mortality league tables: Question what they tell you—and how useful they are. *British Medical Journal* 2003; 326(7393): 777–8.

257 U.S. Department of Health and Human Services. *Healthy People 2010: Understanding and Improving Health (2nd Ed.)*. Washington, DC, US Government Printing Office, 2000.

258 US Department of Health and Human Services. *Healthy People 2000: national Health Promotion and Disease Prevention Objectives 1991*. Darby, PA, DIANE Publishing, 2004.

259 Boufford J, Lee P. *Health Policies for the 21st Century: Challenges and Recomendations for the U.S. Department of Health and Human Services*.

260 Office of State Drug Policy and Meth Coordinator. *Methamphetamine in Minnesota: A Report on the Impact of One Illicit Drug*. Saint Paul, Minnesota, Minnesota Department of Health, 2008.

261 Crawford B, Lilo S, Stone P, Yates A. *Review of the Quality, Safety and Management of Maternity Services in the Wellington region*. Wellington, Ministry of Health, 2008.

262 Department of Health. *Promoting Health in Hong Kong: A Strategic Framework for Prevention and Control of Non-communicable Diseases*. Hong Kong, Hong Kong Special Administrative Region of China Government, 2008.

263 Scullion P. Effective dissemination strategies. *Nurse Res* 2002; 10(1): 65–77.

264 Kothari A, Birch S, Charles C. "Interaction" and research utilisation in health policies and programs: Does it work?. *Health Policy* 2005; 71(1): 117–25.

265 Dobbins M, Ciliska D, Cockerill R, Barnsley J, et al. A framework for the dissemination and utilization of research for health-care policy and practice. *Online J Knowl Synth Nurs* 2002; 9: 7.

266 Rogers E. *Diffusion of Innovations*. New York, The Free Press, 1995.

267 Vingilis E, Hartford K, Schrecker T, et al. Integrating knowledge generation with knowledge diffusion and utilization: A case study analysis of the consortium for applied research and evaluation in mental health. *Canadian Journal of Public Health* 2003; 94(6): 468–71.

268 West E, Barron D, Dowsett J, Newton J. Hierarchies and cliques in the social networks of health care professionals: implications for the design of dissemination strategies. *Social Science and Medicine* 1999; 48(5): 633–46.

269 Stead M, Hastings G, Eadie D. The challenge of evaluating complex interventions: a framework for evaluating media advocacy. *Health Education Research* 2002; 17(3): 351–64.

270 Department of Health. *NHS Next Stage Review: Our Vision for Primary and Community Care: What it Means for Patients and the Public.* London, National Health Service, 2008.

271 Department of Health. *NHS Next Stage Review: Our Vision for Primary and Community Care: What it means for GP and Practice Staff.* London, NHS, 2008.

272 Department of Health. *NHS Next Stage Review: Our Vision for Primary and Community Care: What it Means for Nurses, Midwives, Health Visitors and AHPs.* London, National Health Service.

273 Department of Health. *NHS Next Stage Review: Our Vision for primary and Community Care: What it Means for Local Government.* London, National Health Service, 2008.

274 Lord Darzi. Quality and the NHS next stage review. *Lancet* 2008; 371(9624): 1563–4.

275 The NHS Confederation. *Briefing: High-Quality Care for All.* London, The NNHS Confederation, 2008.

276 Berwick DM. A transatlantic review of the NHS at 60. *British Medical Journal* 2008; 337(jul17_1): a838.

277 Carvel J. NHS review: patient choice at heart of health service revolution. The Guardian. 2008 30 June.

Index